The Top 10 Traits

of

Highly Resilient People

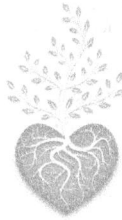

Created and Compiled
by Andrea Pennington, MD, C.Ac.

Featuring stories by:

Berit Bosdal — Helga "Gegga" Birgisdóttir

Sarah K Brandis — Alexsa Covelli

Bruce Cryer — Eric Gerson

Susan Edwards — Rob Goddard

Cynthia J Harrison — Malin Hedlund

Lene Kirk — Deri Llewellyn-Davies

Willow McIntosh — Catherine McLeod

Andrea Pennington, M.D., C.Ac.

Joana Soares — Gerd Stautland

Jill Stocker, D.O. — Åshild Tilrem

Mona Winbrant — Ann Marie Wyrsch

MAKE YOUR MARK GLOBAL

MAKE YOUR MARK GLOBAL PUBLISHING, LTD

USA & Monaco

The Top 10 Traits of Highly Resilient People © 2019 Andrea Pennington, MD, C. Ac.

Published by Make Your Mark Global Publishing, LTD

Book cover design: Andrea Danon & Stefan Komljenović of Art Biro Network www.artbiro.ba

Library of Congress Cataloging-in-Publication Data

Library of Congress Control Number: 2017917382

The Top 10 Traits of Highly Resilient People

Publisher: Make Your Mark Global, LTD

Fernley, Nevada

Pages - 362

Trade Paperback ISBN 978-1-7341526-2-3

Ebook ISBN 978-1-7341526-3-0

Subjects: Psychology

Summary: In The Top 10 Traits of Highly Resilient People Dr. Andrea Pennington presents 21 real life stories of people from various backgrounds and cultures who have dug deep within themselves to overcome, bounce back and move forward after facing difficult and even life threatening circumstances. What these stories all have in common is how they prove that the traits of resilience can be built and expanded with intention so that we can thrive after trauma, and experience more growth than we thought possible. There is great hope and inspiration to be found here.

MAKE YOUR MARK GLOBAL PUBLISHING, LTD

USA

The Top 10 Traits of Highly Resilient People © 2019 Andrea Pennington

For information on bulk purchase orders of this book or to book Dr. Andrea to speak at your event or on your program,

call +33 06 12 74 77 09 or send an email to Booking@AndreaPennington.com

Also Compiled or Co-authored by Andrea Pennington

Magic and Miracles

Life After Trauma

Time to Rise

Turning Points / Vendepunkter

Heart to Heart: The Path to Wellness

Resilience Through Yoga and Meditation

DEDICATION

This book is lovingly dedicated to all of the beautiful souls
who have experienced burnout, loss, illness and trauma

May this book remind you that
you are stronger than you know

May you find inspiration and hope
while reclaiming your resilience

Preface

The book you hold in your hands is a collection of very generous, honest stories from courageous authors. Each of them has opened up their heart to bring you insight into what led them out of pain, confusion and breakdowns into their present lives which are full of beauty, joy and light. These stories of resilience demonstrate that we are stronger than we know!

Because our authors are from a variety of countries and we are publishing these stories in English you may notice that the spelling of words is sometimes in British English and sometimes in American English, depending on the author's country of origin. You'll also see that some phrases they use are unknown to you, as they are not always direct translations from their mother tongue.

In light of the fact that many of our authors are not native English speakers, our team of editors has worked hard to make each story clear and full of the impact the author intended. It is our sincere hope that we have done their compelling stories justice and that you will be moved and inspired by them.

If you'd like to hear the authors in their own voice and watch as they provide context and color to how they decided that this is the time to break their silence I invite you to visit www.MakeYourMarkGlobal.com to watch interviews conducted by the book's publisher, Dr. Andrea Pennington.

Contents

Introduction

The topic of resilience is one that has fascinated me since childhood. Growing up with a family physician in the home, my mother, I often heard stories of devastation, loss, illness and death on a regular basis. It wasn't that my mother brought her work home with her, it was because I worked as 'Office Manager' in her medical practice by the age of 13. I was good at filing, answering phones and making copies of patient records. And I was really good at listening.

Long before health coaches existed, my mom functioned as one. She wasn't the typical medical doctor you may think of who spends only a few minutes in consultation before handing out prescriptions and quickly rushing on to the next patient. My mother, or Dr. P, as she was fondly called, spent an extraordinary amount of time with her patients. She knew their family histories inside and out, and she knew about their dreams and wishes as much as she knew the levels of their blood pressure, fasting blood sugar and cholesterol.

The time my mother spent counseling her patients, whether in the office or on hospital rounds, amounted to intensive coaching on lifestyle and behavior modification. And her guidance on changing one's mindset and her providing psychology hacks made her the go-to doc to get your life, relationships and health straightened out.

Dr. P firmly believed in her patients' abilities to heal, recover and even thrive in the face of illness. She knew how to draw out the innate strengths of her patients, how to shift their mindset to more positive and empowering thought processes and how to encourage them through their darkest hours. She knew how to inspire her patients to never give up, to persevere and to be kind to themselves in the face of tragedy. My mother was the first expert I knew who could coach people to become more resilient.

She knew how to do all of this, and more, because life had delivered to her devastating circumstances that forced her to develop those qualities for herself. Growing up in British Guyana in the 30's, my mom was the youngest of 5 children born to an extraordinary, independent businesswoman. My maternal grandmother inherited a soap factory and by all counts was a strong entrepreneur and all around force to be reckoned with. With a tall, imposing stature and confident tone of voice, she was respected and well revered in Guyana.

Sadly, my grandmother had type II diabetes, and in her mid forties, when my mother was only 11 years old, she succumbed to the disease. My mother watched her powerful, loving mom become bedridden and eventually die from complications of the disease. It left an intense wound inside her.

Because my mom's father was not in the picture, her siblings took charge of the business, the estate and my mom's schooling. They were shocked to hear that in her early twenties my mother intended to move to England to study nursing. She was met with horrified remarks about how inappropriate nursing would be, after all, she would have to examine naked people.

But the experience of watching her mother die a painful death at home inspired my mother to pursue a career in the health field at all costs. When she was midway through her nursing degree, mom says she was shocked to find out that type II diabetes was not only preventable but also a treatable disease that didn't have to end in premature death. It was then that she became determined to use her knowledge and life force to never let anyone die of a preventable disease. She took up a healing crusade that would become her legacy.

When she immigrated to the United States a few years later and worked in a local hospital in Sacramento, she discovered that American physicians were not as civil as their British counterparts. In particular, she was dismayed with the harsh way they spoke down to nurses and lorded their degrees over them. Never one to tolerate condescending attitudes, my feisty mother decided to go to medical school.

So, with three small children at home, she applied for medical school, and got in. Despite her age (she was in her mid thirties by then) and despite being recently divorced, she decided to stand up to the patriarchal medical system to demonstrate how a physician could be compassionate and not arrogant.

I admired the way my pint-sized mother commanded the attention of prominent social and medical personnel along her career, all while being the compassionate, health advocate for her patients. Being a woman of color in the medical profession required that she stand her ground on a number of occasions, to get the same privileges her white male counterparts received. She was driven and dedicated. And during that period of time it is safe to say that she dealt with stress on a constant basis.

Though her drive and being a single mother meant that she would be working outside of our home 5 days a week and some weekends, she also taught me the importance of rest, self-care and play. Mom understood personally how the 10 resilience traits outlined in this book could create a stress resistant personality and lead to a vibrant, meaningful life. She lived these principles, made them her personal mantras and taught them with such gusto that her patients knew many of them by heart.

These resilience traits saved my mother from falling into despair and depression when she lost her mother at such a young age. They empowered her to take on an advanced degree despite facing racism and ageism while raising three kids as a single mother. These resilience traits even helped her keep dementia at bay for decades longer than anyone in her family. She became a physician at the ripe age of 40 and continued her crusade to nurture, coach and heal patients all the way up until she was nearly 70 years old. We even joined forces for a few years when I ran an integrative health center and holistic spa shortly after I finished my medical training.

From being mindfully tuned into the body, becoming aware of genetic and lifestyle influences on health, taking a positive mindset and perspective on recovery, and mixing them with a healthy dose of optimism, perseverance, and a determination to fulfill an inspiring purpose, my mother epitomized the Highly Resilient Person. Through her willful example, and those you'll read in this book, I'm confident that you can become one, too.

What I learned about resilience from the years I shadowed my mother at her medical office was reinforced in medical school, my residency training and the last two decades of working professionally as an integrative physician, healer and mentor. In addition to my conventional medical degree I received certification in acupuncture as well as Age Management Medicine, neurofeedback, nutrition therapy, trauma recovery and positive psychology.

Looking at our health, emotional wellbeing and relationships from multiple perspectives often requires multiple disciplines to manage them, and I'm grateful that my background has afforded me the ability to see health from many angles. I have since had the privilege of accompanying thousands of patients on their healing journeys and witnessing their often miraculous recoveries using an integrative and holistic approach. From terrifying diagnoses like cancer, multiple sclerosis and Alzheimer's dementia, to obesity, depression and fibromyalgia, my exposure to the cause and cure of illness and disease has run the gamut.

In all my years of practicing medicine, leading retreats and teaching workshops, I have faithfully continued in the steps of my mother by bringing focused attention, compassion and plenty of face time to my patients to dive into their health, their past medical histories and their early life experiences. The integrative and holistic approach to wellness I use has allowed me to guide patients toward self-healing in many cases, and accelerated recovery using conventional therapies in most others. Building resilience has become the cornerstone of my medical practice and psychological coaching.

Through my professional connection to doctors, therapists and healers around the world, I have now been exposed to even more cases of people who have put these traits to work as they recovered from burnout, stress-induced illness and even while overcoming the lasting physical and emotional effects of exposure to toxic or traumatic experiences in childhood. While the resilience research is quite extensive, most lay people are unaware of the real world applications of the clinical data. I am happy to report that the true stories presented in this book represent authentic examples of how resilience is built, reinforced and relied upon in real life. I will share with you the latest research findings throughout the book which will show you that these are trustworthy and aim-worthy traits to pursue with actionable exercises you can implement on your own.

Defining resilience

Resilience is a well-defined term in science, psychology and technology. It is defined as an individual's ability to adapt in the face of adverse conditions. In ecological terms, it is the capacity of an ecosystem to recover from perturbations. In organizations and groups, it is the ability of a system to withstand changes in its environment and still function.

A resilient person is often described as being able to bounce back after a tragedy, illness, injury or recover after a setback. Being resilient usually brings to mind terms such as flexible, adaptable, durable, and of strong character.

Resilience is an inborn capacity

We are each born with an internal program for resilience. Modern psychological research concludes that no matter the challenges we face, we have an inborn capacity to adapt to and recover from life's setbacks, illnesses, injuries and accidents. According to medical science, ancient wisdom traditions and even a review of ancient philosophical literature, experts across the millennia have documented that each of us is born with the inherent potential to live a meaningful, happy and healthy life, even in the face of serious adversity.

For most of us, unless there was significant birth trauma, a problematic pregnancy, or an inborn genetic disorder we are born in a state of wellbeing. All of our organ systems are poised for a healthy life, full of the ability to weather the various storms of life with resilience and grace. We are born with the natural tendency to thrive. This is a lifelong tendency.

Just as children bounce back after sickness and surgery, we adults can do the same. The innate biological wisdom for homeostasis and recovery can be tapped right now to recover from illness, injury and disease. Just as children change activities, hobbies and 'best friends' with ease, we adults can change the course of our lives from humdrum to rapturous with little resistance. In fact, we can be dancing, frolicking and playing for decades to come. We are programmed for resilience.

The 5 Elements of Chinese Philosophy

My mother also introduced me to Traditional Chinese Medicine and acupuncture while I was in medical school. I was inspired by the beauty and elegance of Chinese medical philosophy, which points to how we each can enjoy ageless vitality and optimal wellbeing throughout our lifespan. It's about allowing for and optimizing our life to return harmony to our energies.

The ancient Chinese philosophy and the Taoist concepts of the 5 elements along with acupuncture and qigong have truly been a blessing in my life to help understand our personal and Universal energy. According to Traditional Chinese Medicine (TCM), we can renew our vitality and return to a natural state of wholeness and wellness when we live in accordance with our true nature and the flow of nature around us. We each carry an energetic blueprint for optimal wellbeing, happiness and success. This energy imprint dictates how our body, mind and heart naturally integrate to make us whole beings for a long, healthy life of active, vibrant living.

The dynamic life force energy, or 'qi' in Chinese, flows through the sky, earth, our bodies and our surroundings naturally. Where this energy flows, life flourishes. When this life force energy circulates harmoniously through all of our body's channels — or meridians — we can remain healthy and vital for a long, bountiful life. Even when life presents us with illness or injuries, the flow of life force energy enables us to quickly recover. We have an innate ability to bounce back even stronger than ever from illness, injury, shock or trauma.

All of us, both women and men, have a mix of *yin* and *yang* energy. We are made with this fundamental polarity between receptive and aggressive flow. An excess of one or the other is what can lead to *dis-ease*. When we recognize that the human body is meant to return to a state of wholeness and vitality after intense periods of work or stress, it becomes imperative that we consider the many ways that we block our natural inclination for repair and rejuvenation.

At a cellular level, right down to our DNA, we can impact our physical and emotional health as well as our ability to recover from stress, illness and injury. We influence our own wellbeing by honoring our own energy needs, respecting the cycles of life and the rhythms of the seasons and days. Rather than trying to force ourselves to live up to unrealistic external standards, which are often an unattainable and unhealthy, we can learn more about our inherent energy, what allows us to refuel and recharge and ensure that we take part in activities that engage a deeper sense of our being.

The TCM system explains that when we allow our natural energy signature to inform and guide our lifestyle we can live wholly, fully and resiliently. In the Chinese medical view of the human body-mind, we are a microcosm or mini-version of the macrocosm of the entire universe and nature. Just as nature recovers after hurricanes, droughts and volcanic eruptions, when we experience setbacks, illnesses or bumps on our journey through life, they need not derail us entirely. Our own natural forces can bring us back to wellness and set us back on the course to optimal wellbeing and the pursuit of our highest ideals. This is what resilience is all about.

The Chinese have documented this natural ability for over 2,500 years, and now is the time for you to master it as well. You have the potential to become the master of your whole life to enjoy optimal wellbeing of body, mind, spirit, environment and relationships.

To get a sense of how the 5 elements of Chinese Medicine influence your resilience, please visit www.TheVitalityTest.com. There you will find a free online questionnaire developed by my colleague Nick Haines of the Five Institute. Taking the assessment will show you which of the 5 Chinese elements are your dominant influences: Water, Wood, Metal, Earth, Fire. Take the Vitality Test to learn more about what makes you brilliant and vulnerable to stress and how the 5 elements can be helpful in building resilience.

How we deplete our capability to recover

While we are each born with the inherent capacity for resilience, we can, however, become overwhelmed by the drama, trauma and stress in our lives. Our innate vitality code directs several body systems to return us to a state of wellbeing. But prolonged exposure to stressful situations with inadequate resources for coping, managing and diffusing the physiological stress response can overwhelm the body's ability to recover. It can even lead to considerable damage to multiple organ systems.

Overworked bodies, overloaded schedules, and overwhelmed minds use up our vital energy and can leave us feeling exhausted and fatigued. Your vital life force energy can become weak, stuck or sluggish as a result of not living in harmony with your natural energy flow.

For example, not eating healthy food, drinking too much alcohol, or engaging in unhealthy behaviors, relationships and even toxic careers can cause your energy to become depleted or stagnant. When this happens, we experience dis-ease in a variety of forms. We may become sick, tired or depressed, and devoid of joy or passion.

Fortunately, our bodies, including our brains, have incredible capacity for recovery and rejuvenation. There is a reliable path to vitality, purpose and fulfillment which incorporates the well regarded and well researched domains of resilience, neuroscience and positive psychology. The principles of these clinical domains are well represented in the stories of recovery in this book.

My burnout breakthrough

Despite my mother having three children, dealing with sexism and racism in the early part of her medical career, and working really hard, I never saw her drop from exhaustion nor suffer from burnout. Looking back I can see that all of her self-care routines, dancing, listening to the music of her homeland, and gardening were her ways of honoring her own energy type.

Early in my career, I strove to fit into the mold that the media and medical society put me into, without respect for my innate nature it nearly drove me into the ground. The first time I experienced burnout, it hit me hard. I was in my early thirties and had a lot of anxiety, fear, depression and confusion in my head, in addition to physical weakness. I struggled to get out of bed in the morning, I felt emotionally drained and I lost my motivation at work. I felt totally lost, running on autopilot, battling with imposter syndrome.

Because I had previously been so passionate, enthusiastic with my job, I became curious to know where my mojo had gone. And I saw the same thing in many of my clients — from overworked parents and caregivers, to entrepreneurs, highly sensitive coaches, and empathic healers. I started to ask, "why do some highly functional executives, parents or superstars thrive despite high stress and some succumb to burnout and exhaustion?"

I was given a referral to a well-known therapist. He was known for treating high-powered executives and influential people on Capitol Hill in Washington, DC. During our initial session he told me that he thought my case would be easy to fix based on certain traits I already possessed and those he could help me build.

He told me one thing that drove me to research resilience and recovering from burnout. He said, "Andrea you need to become FAT. Flexible, adaptable and tolerant." He explained that these were a few traits of highly resilient people, the types of people who run countries, own large multinational companies, and live as high-performing megastars. He told me that building up resilience could give me more internal peace and even greater productivity.

So, I began my study of burnout, resilience and recovery. Over the years my research led me to add to the list several more characteristics of resilience which I present to you in *The Top 10 Traits of Highly Resilient People.* I'm now more mindful of my tendency to take on projects that won't deplete me. And I'm better at setting boundaries to prevent me from overworking.

How resilience impacts our wellbeing

If balance and wholeness represent our natural state why do some people bounce back easier than others? Why do some rise after defeat rather than wither into obscurity? Why do siblings born into the same families with similar exposures sometimes grow into completely opposite adults? Why do some victims of abuse become abusers as adults while their siblings, who also suffered abuse, become rescuers? What makes one child respond to a demanding, critical parent with perfectionism while another withdraws and becomes an underachiever?

It turns out that innate qualities of personality also influence how we perceive, interpret, and label our experiences. Throughout this book you will learn how to reinterpret, re-label and empower yourself to become more resilient and robust than ever before. Our mental attitude and focus also impact our ability to recover from setbacks. by reading the real life stories presented in this book you'll see how you can adopt new ways of thinking and being which will enhance your resilience factors.

Recovering from and preventing burnout

This book has been inspired by the thousands of people I've encountered over the last decade who've experienced health challenges such as chronic fatigue, fibromyalgia, lupus, depression and anxiety all due to excessive stress. Some of the stress was caused by emotional and physical abuse, some was caused by taking care of sick relatives or special needs children, and some was simply due to overwork.

One of the end points we see as a result of living with excessive stress, is a wearing away of our resilience resources. Ultimately, if we do not release stress, replenish our energy and maintain a healthy lifestyle, we may end up in burnout.

Burnout is defined as the progressive process of physical, emotional & mental exhaustion. It is caused by long-term exposure to stressful, emotionally demanding situations. The symptoms of burnout burnout like overwhelm, chronic fatigue, depression and anxiety are usually associated with work (like in the healing & helping professionals, teachers, entrepreneurs, CEOs,) but burnout is also seen in caregivers of all kinds like parents in general and those with children having special needs, caregivers for elderly or sick, as I share in Chapter 4.

Research shows that people who are susceptible to burnout were initially highly motivated and enthusiastic about their work/role, but over time stressful conditions wore away their emotional and physical reserves, replacing them with disillusionment, cynicism and all out depletion of their motivation. In the past we could work our butts off and hustle hard, relying on caffeine or energy drinks and resting on the weekends. But the pace of our lifestyle keeps pouring demands and desires upon us. Our time is a limited resource, but the demands keep coming. The old way of life is not sustainable. The combination of dependence or addiction to cope or keep up, overwork and overwhelm wreak havoc on our physical and emotional wellbeing. Millions of people realize that the constant hustle does not lead to satisfaction or fulfillment, at worst it can lead to an early death, and at the very least poor physical health and mental illness.

Rates of burnout and exhaustion are at an all-time high — and given our lifestyle those rates will continue to go higher. We are more aware than ever of the dire need for recovery from stress, trauma and everyday life trauma to keep families and whole communities together. Our individual and collective resilience is needed to recover from burnout and to prevent it from happening again. It's time to turn it around, before it's too late. Now is the time to find a new way to live and thrive, a new way to defeat stress, renew our energy and replenish our willpower. It's time for us all to develop more resilience.

The structure of this book

Each chapter of the book covers one trait of the top traits of highly resilient people. After a brief explanation of the trait, one or more personal stories are presented by contributing authors. You will be inspired to investigate and improve the deepest aspects of your personality, the ones not taught in school and mostly reserved for psychotherapy offices, to help you enhance recovery, rewire your brain and find the deepest meaning in life.

It is my sincere wish that this book inspires and empowers you to reactivate your innate vitality code and build even more resilience.

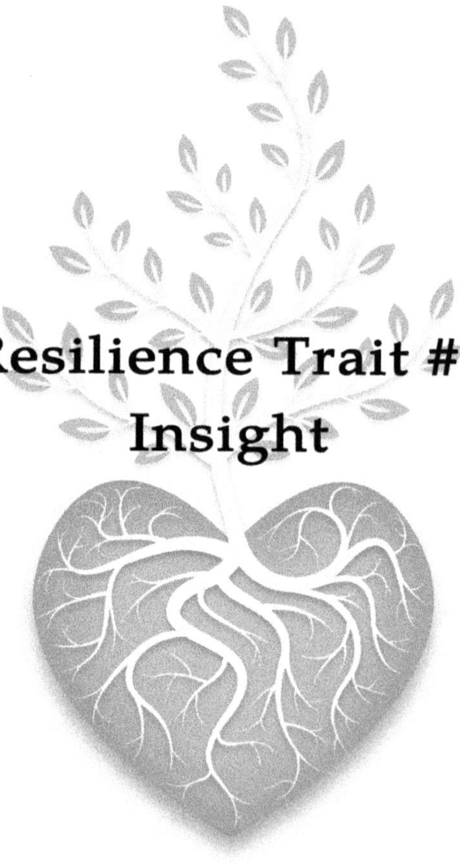

Resilience Trait #1
Insight

The number one trait of highly resilient people is insight. Insight is all about self-awareness and emotional intelligence. These are key resources which build resilience. Insight empowers you to rebound from setbacks, breakdowns and burnout more gracefully and increases the likelihood that you will come back stronger after recovering from overwhelm and overdoing. Part of self-awareness, or insight involves increasing your emotional intelligence. This helps you recognize your own emotional triggers that make you feel stressed or deplete your energy. This type of intelligence also helps you identify the feelings other people may be experiencing.

To develop a stress resistant personality we begin by addressing a potential lack of insight, a lack of self-awareness. The absence of awareness is also defined as ignorance — but this does not mean stupidity, it simply implies 'not knowing.' Not being aware of or denying your own mental and emotional makeup and what you require to thrive will leave you at risk of burnout, illness and even premature death.

Developing emotional intelligence and insight into your feelings while also becoming open, curious and actively investigating your makeup will build resilience. More than that, developing greater self-awareness is the foundation of a life of peace, fulfillment, joy, ease and flow.

Understanding yourself, who you really are and what makes you tick is where you begin to align your actions with your true nature. And this is the first step to activating your innate vitality code — the body's natural blueprint for recovery, resilience and restoration. When you live in alignment with your authentic self and your core values you allow your innate vitality code to turn on the body's rest and recovery systems. And it helps you build a stress-resistant personality.

Without insight we tend to walk around blindly, reacting to life based on old programs, rather than tuning into greater wisdom in the present moment. Without insight you stay in self-denial and unhealthy lifestyles. Without awareness of your strengths and limits you stay stuck in self-doubt.

With self-awareness and insight into who you really are you can stop comparing your life, talents, burdens, and outcomes against anything or anyone outside of you. Instead you get clear about your own system for wellbeing, your symptoms, and your stress triggers and you can create your own personalized recovery plan that works for YOU.

As I mentioned in the Introduction, one way you can increase self awareness and insight is by taking Vitality Test, developed by my colleague Nick Haines of the Five Institute. This free online questionnaire will show you which of the 5 Chinese elements are your dominant influences: Water, Wood, Metal, Earth, Fire. Visit www.TheVitalityTest.com to learn more about what makes you brilliant and vulnerable to stress and how the 5 elements can be helpful in building resilience. This will be useful as you read the stories presented in this book.

Our first personal story, by Gerd Stautland, demonstrates the power of developing insight into our emotional makeup and our triggers. Gerd is a compassionate teacher who lived most of her life blind to the source of intense suffering she experienced in relationships. Well into adulthood she discovered how a situation in early childhood created a deep emotional wound. This new insight into her past led her to explore healing modalities that ultimately set her free from that old pain and inspired her to transform her life.

Then a story by Åshild Tilrem, a licensed critical care nurse, shows us that while we are all born resilient, certain life circumstances that shape our beliefs can steer us away from our natural ability to recover from stress. Her story details how the mind-body connection can provide us with clues when we are going against our nature and leading toward a stressful, disease provoking state. She explains beautifully how we can choose empowering thoughts that lift up our mood and enhance our wellbeing.

Thorn Surrenders to Rose
by Gerd Stautland

She saw the BACK of her father through the glass door, walking away from her. Leaving her alone at the hospital among strangers for 6 weeks. She was in horrible pain with kidney stones. The strange smell of the hospital. The nurses and doctors dressed in all white. The white and very stiff bedclothes against her skin. The cold metal cot, like a cage.

The silence.

She was 22 months old, far away from home, from her mum and her sister.

She was paralyzed. The desperate scream that grew inside her did not come. Something died in her, and she learned to be silent, to not speak up for herself, and not to trust anyone.

This is my first memory. It impacted my life on a profound level.

I grew up on an island on the west coast of Norway, surrounded by high mountains, deep fjords, lakes and forests.

This wild and beautiful nature became my best friend early on.

My mother came from the middle part of Norway, where the mentality seemed to be "light", carefree and joyful. My father was born and grew up on the same island as me. Some will say that the mentality in this part of Norway was very much characterized by Christianity, judgement, prejudice, shame and guilt.

Most of my life I felt as I was dragged between these two mentalities, as if two imaginary people or voices were inside of me constantly fighting for my attention.

I call these two imaginary "characters" Rose and Thorn.

I remember myself as a lonely and quiet child, longing to be seen, heard, loved, and to belong. I never felt good, smart or pretty enough. My self-confidence was low. Most of the time I was controlled by the Thorn voice inside of me.

Inside I had a big, open wound, but I did not have a clue where it came from.

Throughout all my childhood I struggled with horrible stomach pains. No doctor could find anything wrong with me, physically.

On the other side, I was a very curious child, never afraid of trying and learning new things and skills, always searching for new adventures. I took a lot of chances. My father called me foolhardy. Music, needlework and sports were my biggest interests, and playing with these I had a lot of fun, accompanied by the Rose voice in me!

I was an easy victim when a grownup man paid attention to me. At 17 years old I became pregnant. With no support from the father, I ended up in a home for single mothers in Oslo.

When my contractions started, the caretaker of the home brought me to THAT hospital, the same as I was left 15 years ago!

He followed me to the front desk, turned his BACK to me and left. I was terrified to death of what was in front of me, feeling lonelier than ever. But after 64 hours my beautiful daughter was born. I loved her from the first moment, and I remember thinking to myself: "I have enough love for both of us!"

Eight months later I moved back to the west coast and started at the Teacher College. Good years followed, and I had a lot of fun. Rose came by often. However, Thorn was never far away. He could pop up in the most unexpected ways and times, and feelings could sneak up on me and catch me in seconds. It was like a scab on a wound that was torn up, again and again. I was so tired of this Thorn but I didn't have a clue how to get rid of him!

After finishing my studies, I got a job as a teacher in the northernmost town in Norway, very far away from home. At 22 years old, alone with a daughter of 4 ½ years, who just wanted to go home to her grandma, this was a very tough situation! Thorn was very present in this time and controlled most of my days.

A colleague at school was very caring and showed me attention. He lit up our days, and soon we were a couple. Two years later we married and moved back to the south of Norway. We were blessed with another beautiful daughter, whom we all loved very much.

But my internal struggles continued. Rose and Thorn were in constant conflict. I could not love myself, and from this "empty cup" I had not much to give. I was not able to connect fully from my heart and share my inner life. My internal conflicts became external.

No one could fill the big, dark, empty hole in me. The lack of self-confidence, the feeling of loneliness and disconnection. My daughters were my biggest comfort. My husband and I divorced.

In the years that followed I went into several relationships, hoping and believing that THIS time I had met the ONE that could meet all my needs, that could heal my big wound. But I continued in the same pattern, no lessons learned. Rose and Thorn always fought about my attention, and very often Thorn won!

I unconsciously developed strategies to control, myself and my partner, afraid of being left. I didn't see how this way of clinging to the control limited me, and us! I built up distance so it shouldn't be so painful to distinguish. The distance made it more painful to be together.

The Law of Attraction worked perfectly each time — of course I was left! Or I left, because I believed that my partner would leave me anyway, better to get over with!

One day, back in 2000, I met my eldest daughter for a dinner out in Oslo. We had a really good time together. Outside the restaurant we said goodbye, hugged each other and everything was fine. After walking away in opposite directions, I just turned around, and then I saw her BACK.

I started trembling, and a tremendous sadness and grief overwhelmed me, the tears flew down my cheeks. At this moment I started to realize the context of my struggles through life when it came to saying goodbye to people, to see people leaving me, even for a short time or distance!

Could it connect with my memory of THE BACK from the hospital in 1956? I asked my father about this experience, and he sadly admitted that he left me two times in the hospital. The second one when he came to pick me up after six weeks. I was not ready to leave when he came, the doctor wanted to take some extra tests. My father went away to "fix" something in Oslo while he was waiting. When, at last, he came to pick me up, I showed no signs of recognition. It was as if my face were carved in stone, he told me.

Then I started to understand more of my pain, my big wound, the feeling of loneliness and disconnection in life, my emotions related to saying goodbye. I understood why I couldn't trust anyone fully and my fear of tying very tight ties, but I didn't know how to heal.

Thorn was still very present in my life and he was always fighting with Rose. She always wanted to dance, sing and have fun. Others saw me as a strong and independent woman, fixing everything on my own. Inside I was vulnerable and often felt lonely and not belonging, kind of "homeless".

I went into a new relationship, and guess what? The same old story happened! Still no lesson learned! In 2005 I was left again. This time I fell into the deepest darkness of my life! The pain was intolerable, it was like an iron claw in my heart! I could not sleep, eat or work. I could barely breathe.

I escaped to my cabin in the mountains, well accompanied by Thorn. Nature has always been the best place for me to be alone with my loneliness, as it was this time too. I cried out all my tears. I lived in this total darkness for about four months.

One beautiful morning in the mountains, lying in bed, with the most amazing view to the high mountains, I had a glimpse of light. I realized that I had to choose: To break through this darkness and connect with Rose again, or to let Thorn check me and break myself totally down.

I decided to search for Rose again!

On this day I went for a long walk, and for the first time in months, I started to see the beauty around me. I started to smell the sweet fragrance of heather that is so strong in autumn in the mountains. I heard the birds singing and felt the soft wind and the sun on my skin.

I felt a glimpse of life again! And I knew for sure that this day was the first day of my new life. I was ready to surrender Thorn to Rose!

My daughters were very caring and supporting during this time, and I realized that THEY, and my life were reasons to live for! All the previous times when I ended up in the dark place I used to start a physical, external project, such as refurbishing my homes, building my own house, etc, just to show myself and everybody that I managed all by myself.

This time I decided to start an internal project, to go inside, connect with myself and try to heal my wound.

As this very special and important day of my life faded out, I found Rose again, and I made a deal with her: She promised to support me and stay by my side.

A long journey began. How? The "landscape" of self-healing and self-development were unknown to me. Some days later, on my way back home, I stopped in a town. I passed a bookstore and was really drawn into it. And there, after walking by the bookshelves for a while, Louise Hay smiled so beautifully to me and "said": You can heal your life!

WOW! I knew immediately that this was an answer to my questions! This book gave me the best start on my new journey. New books were bought: *The Power of your Thoughts* by Wayne Dyer, *The Seven Spiritual Laws of Success* by Deepak Chopra, and *Ask and it Shall Be Given* by Esther and Jerry Hicks, to name a few.

I read every book I put my hands on, went to courses, retreats, to events. I learned EFT, (Emotional Freedom Technique) and Hypnotherapy. Using the tools and techniques on myself and experiencing the healing power of them and my energies shifted. I was no longer so vulnerable, the old wound was not triggered in the same way as before.

Thorn had lost a lot of his power!

I realized that my life was my own responsibility; physically, emotionally and mentally. I learned the power of forgiveness, and how it set me free. I moved from the victim role to "The Captain" of my own life.

After a while I started to feel a burning desire to share my tools with others. I became a Therapist and set up my own business. At this point in time I was still a school teacher, and I tried to teach the children at school the powerful tool of EFT but was stopped by some parents. "Alternative Treatments are not allowed in school," they claimed.

One year later I decided to quit my job as a teacher. The rigid nature of the school system diverged too strongly from my innermost values. I was unstoppable. I wanted to learn more and heal all. I wanted Thorn to surrender to Rose! I wanted to have fun, to be loving, joyful, free and accepting Rose to be my "partner" for the rest of my life. A new happy and healthy life in flow was what I aimed for. The connection to myself and who I AM got stronger. I had travelled from my head to my heart. My life was transformed.

In December 2016, a Facebook post popped up on my newsfeed, and it really caught my attention. It was about the European Transformational Teachers Gathering, ETTG, hosted by Steinar Ditlefsen, Spain, April 2017. I knew immediately that this was something I wanted to attend, and I ordered my ticket straight away.

Honestly, I didn't really know what I was attending, but at this time I had started to listen more to my intuition. I went alone, knowing nobody, except Steinar. Sitting in the breakfast room the first day I had a very strong experience. Two beautiful women entered the room. Their loving energies and feminine power were so strong, they nearly blew me away! I could really feel a connection with these beautiful souls!

And after breakfast, entering the room for the event, set in the most beautiful palm garden, I felt surrendered with such a warm, loving and including atmosphere that I had never experienced before! I felt at home. I felt connected. Soon I came to know some beautiful souls, all with the purpose to help other people live better life. There was no judgement, no competition, I felt totally accepted, as ME!

Some of the speakers generously offered their programs for free, and curious as I am, I went into all of them. I learned a lot, practiced a lot, found my purpose, my mission, my "drive". I learned to love and accept myself, I found more happiness, joy and freedom. I became my own best friend. Some of the people that I met on ETTG have impacted my life on a deep level. Working with their programs, attending their events and connecting with others opened some new doors for me, and helped me to heal even more. I got very conscious of how our energies impact our lives, and energy work is what I have become passionate about. Some of the missing bricks in my life puzzle fell into place!

I "set my days" with yoga, meditations and exercises. I check that my energies are in flow. I nourish my body in the best way. I spend time in nature every day. I live in the "Abundance room", with an attitude of gratitude. I know hard times will occur, but I now have "tools" to meet them with. I am deeply grateful for all my mentors through life. They have guided me and helped me along this long and winding road that my life has been, to become the person I am today.

Thorn has surrendered to Rose.

It took me 14 years to fully heal my wound. Now I want to help other people who are struggling in life. I want to increase their awareness of how important our energies are for our physical, emotional and mental health. I want to help them to live a happy and healthy life in flow, accepting and loving themselves.

"I greet my day with love in my heart!"

About the Author
Gerd Stautland

Gerd Stautland was a teacher for 34 years, and she loved to work with children. However, in 2010 the school system had become more and more rigid, and diverged too much away from her values, and she was not able to work as a teacher any longer.

Some years before she had a breakdown in her own life, which prompted her to start on her journey of self-development to try to heal her big wound, caused by a trauma from early childhood.

She came across EFT (The Emotional Freedom Technique), and her big interest for energy work was ignited. She is a student of Donna Eden's Energy Medicine and Yvette Taylor's EAM (Energy Alignment Method).

Gerd is now an EFT practitioner and Hypnotherapist. She runs Energy Workshops, and works 1-to-1 with clients to help them raise their energies and release stuck energies so they can live a happier and happier life in more flow.

You find her on the 'Fri Energiflyt' FB page: https://www.facebook.com/frienergiflyt/

We Are Born Resilient
by Åshild Tilrem

Though it was almost twenty years ago, I remember it as
if it were yesterday. I was working as a nurse in the
emergency department in one of the public hospitals in
Norway. Standing in the middle of the emergency room,
ready and waiting to receive another patient from a suicide
attempt, I could already feel the inner tsunami of emotions
flooding me. But I knew I had to stay professional in that
moment, suppressing what I felt. This is something I had
always mastered so perfectly.

As soon as the patient arrived, I immediately recognized
her. It was the same woman I received just a couple of days
before. She was a few years younger than me, a married
mother of two small kids. As her last attempt of ending her
life wasn't successful, she had now decided to swallow a full
box of painkillers in another attempt to escape the world, her
intense pain, and the feeling of despair and hopelessness she
had felt for so long. I could really relate to the pain she must
have felt. I had been struggling myself with suicidal
thoughts since I was 13 years old.

She was laying there in the bed, totally apathetic,
probably disappointed by the fact that she was still
breathing. I took her hand and tried to make eye contact
with her, just to let her know that I saw her and felt her, and
of course informed her about what was going to happen
during the next few minutes. I knew that she was fully

aware of what we had to do to stabilize her medical condition. Still, it always felt like an abuse to force a tube down the throat of a patient in such a deep emotional pain, to pump the stomach to prevent liver damage from the pills she swallowed. After finishing the acute procedures and her physical examination by the doctor, I took her to a patient room for her to rest.

A relentless pursuit for answers

That day in the emergency room I made myself a promise; I should find a solution to help these people *before* they became suicidal. This promise got even stronger when a few years later I graduated as an intensive care nurse and realized how much stigma there was in the medical field when it came to mental illness and suicide attempts. Obviously, there was a clear difference in the way patients were treated depending on the type of attempt committed. If they became critically ill and ended up as an intensive care patient, they were put at the top of the medical hierarchy, compared to those admitted to the psychiatric hospital, who were apparently not worth a penny. For me, every human being deserves to be treated with dignity, respect and kindness, no matter what their story was. Witnessing this unfairness strengthened my deep and genuine desire to help people.

This was when my journey began for real. An endless search for answers to the mystery of health and happiness started, and became my top priority. It became more important than taking care of myself and reacting to the signals my body was trying to show me. Next to my job as a nurse I was literally looking in every corner of the world. I studied several modalities in the healing arts and the alternative medicine field, trying to find the missing links to health and become able to see the whole picture.

Along with this journey I went through several periods of burnout and depression myself; serious infections, loss of my father, two miscarriages, relationship-break up, and in the end I was diagnosed with chronic fatigue syndrome and couldn't leave the bed for weeks and months. It was a huge shock for me and difficult to accept that my body went into total strike and was emotionally torn down. I had always thought that I was quite stress-proof and able to handle crisis situations and deal with difficult emotions. Now it was time to take the messages seriously, listen to my body and learn to practice self-care.

Knowing that there was not much help, support or explanation to get in the western medical system, I quickly realized that I had to be my own doctor and my own psychologist. This conviction became even stronger when a psychiatrist told me I was born depressed and the only solution was to take antidepressants for the rest of my life. Luckily, this "death message" triggered my inner warrior more than tearing me down. So, as soon as I got out of bed and was back on my feet again, my journey continued.

With my holistic-thinking-brain and one foot in both camps, I started my master's degree in public health and dove deep into the topic of alternative treatments for depression and burnout. My curious and inquisitive mind started to ask questions like; why do we get sick, depressed and burnt out initially? Why did some people seem to cope with life struggles better than others and bounce back more quickly? According to the literature the answers lay in resilience, our inner capacity to cope with adversity in life. But, was resilience a gift handed down from above only to some lucky and blessed individuals?

The answer was no.

Being a spiritual person, I had a deep knowing within that we are all born with this inner life force connected to a divine source that makes us naturally resilient, with an innate capacity to heal, transform and survive. Though we are all born with different degrees of physical and psychological vulnerability, we are built to survive! How could a baby otherwise manage to go through the narrow birth channel if it was not equipped with an innate ability to cope with such a trauma? I was also a living proof of that. I was called a "miracle baby" as I was almost strangled with the umbilical cord three times around my neck. I didn't show much in the way of vital signs after being delivered via an urgent caesarean. With an Apgar score of 1-2, the birth team had to initiate an immediate resuscitation. I was intubated and ventilated for the first 15 minutes of my life and put in an incubator for several days, totally separated from my mother, which is a huge trauma for a newborn. Still I grew into a quite functional and capable child. The literature is also full of examples of people who have survived and thrived against all odds.

I started to ask the questions in a different way; if we were all born resilient, what took our resilience away from us? What made us less resilient? Finding answers to these questions has brought me more value than any of the techniques or modalities I have studied. It has blessed me with some life-changing and life-saving insights that have brought me back to more health and wholeness, and which I would love to share with you.

This path of awakening has been like an inner "death and rebirth" process, though the most important insights came during a retreat I attended some years back. I woke up after being in a meditative state and it was as if every cell in my body realized something new at the same time. I had some sudden realizations of truth that left me with infinite hope and inspiration. I got some profound insights that created a huge shift in my consciousness and gave me a new sense of inner peace and clarity. It was just like a veil was gone from my head and everything became transparent. I could see through the illusions we create in our minds. Suddenly I felt there was nothing I needed to worry about any more, if I only understood these two things:

1. How our mind works and how we work as human beings at our deepest level.

2. Life is all about love and connection. Not only connection to ourselves and other people, but connection to God and the higher source of wisdom.

Understanding the mind

With these insights, one of the most important discoveries I had was understanding *how our thoughts* create our reality and experience of life at any moment, separate us from the truth, and create pain and suffering. This understanding has been vital to my health.

Most of our problems, if not every one of them, comes from a "disturbed" mind or "malign" way of thinking, which is a result of our interpretations of our life experiences, our energetic imprints in our DNA and programs we have adopted from our environment from the very first years of our lives, often in a pre-cognitive phase. It is like the original sin. We make conclusions about ourselves and the world from our early life traumas of being abandoned and rejected, and run these programs until we one day wake up and realize that this has nothing to do with who we really are. It is our "toxic" thinking originating from a "toxic" environment.

As Bruce Lipton points out in his book *The Biology of Belief,* our mind is totally habitual and can only play back what it learns. A shocking 90-95 % of our life comes from our programming in the subconscious mind, and most of the time we are playing programs that we have adopted from other people and our "family tree". It is like we "download" a generational software and see life through filters that come from these preconditioned programs and not from our true and authentic self. These patterns become our reality, our everyday language and create our identity, or rather our "false identity". We start to believe that we *are* our thoughts and emotions.

With all the pain and suffering in the environment I grew up in, at some level I thought I was destined to suffer and totally sacrifice myself for the sake of others. I was raised and programmed to be a "people pleaser" and take care of other people's needs before my own. As an adult, this became especially true in my relationships where I had trouble setting good boundaries as I was afraid of hurting anyone. I would end up being depressed and totally drained. When we suppress our own needs and our own authenticity for the sake of others, we are not in alignment with our true essence and the body starts to speak the truth for us.

Learning to really see this mind-body connection has been a pivotal turning point for me. Now, I can immediately sense in every cell of my body when I chose from my own truth and when I'm not controlled by my inherent programs and "toxic" thinking. Every choice we make has an energetic consequence for our body. Choosing the truth makes my body feel more expanded, relaxed and at ease, while doing the opposite weakens me and puts my body into contraction, tension and stress mode. As the spiritual author, Caroline Myss says; "the distance between our head and our heart is what creates *dis-ease*". We are not at ease in ourselves and this creates an underlying stress reaction in our body.

Likewise, living in a chronic condition of unhealthy thinking and not understanding where our feelings are coming from, creates a situation of "dis-ease" in the body. Every human being uses the power of thought to create our own subjective psychological experience from within. We all experience negative thoughts, but it is up to us how we will relate to the content of our thoughts. Before I had this realization I constantly drained myself with the same symphony in my head; *I was not good enough or smart enough. I was doomed to carry the cross of life on my shoulders.* Now, I can easily spot any thoughts that don't serve me and better understand where they originate from. Then, I can replace them with more empowering and nurturing thoughts.

With this awareness, I also started to see that we are all innocent in this "game". There is no reason to blame or judge others as they are operating from their own wounds and "distorted" programming. As a nurse working with other nurses in stressful situations, I could more easily show compassion instead of taking everything personally. I understood that their stress reactions had nothing to do with me. The same was true with my family members. So many times, I felt totally overwhelmed and frustrated about their somewhat infantile emotional reaction patterns. Realizing that this was their own unconscious inner mental programming, I would rather observe the "craziness" and remain calm and relaxed in the situation. It didn't get a grip on me anymore and I stopped reacting with exhaustion. Clearly, having this understanding prevents us from being the "victim" of forces beyond our control.

Love and connection

The second insight I had made me realize the importance of love and connection to all there is. As human beings one of our most essential needs is the need for attachment and connection to other people. We are all social beings and need to feel a sense of belonging. This is a natural part of our human existence. Many of us are carrying blueprints of attachment traumas and emotional neglect from early life (or from our family system), which colors how we perceive the world as adults and relate to other people. Experiences of separation and disconnection live inside us as our lives unfold and prevent us from creating healthy and intimate relationships.

When we are immersed in these beliefs of unworthiness and brokenness originating from these experiences, we reinforce the feeling of separation and loneliness and create an underlying stress situation in the body. Recognizing and understanding how our mind and these beliefs separate and alienate us from each other and from the source, made a huge shift for me. At this retreat, I experienced a moment of total connection to everything and everyone. I saw beyond the illusions of our mind and how a lack of insights and understanding leads to unnecessary pain and suffering. What became clear to me was that everything that puts our body into a stress mode or separates us from the source, will make us less resilient as it disrupts the natural energy flow in the body and disturbs our innate intelligence. We will be more susceptible to burnout and chronic disease.

Being connected to spirit and living from a loving state more than a fear based state, will make us naturally resilient and create more calmness inside. This is our natural state of being beyond our thinking and our bonds to the past. Knowing that we are all part of this divine source of love and recognizing that we can always access this innate health and resilience as soon as we disengage in our personal thinking and reconnect with spirit. This has brought me a new sense of inner peace and freedom and also made me able to support my clients in a more empowering way.

My greatest realization is that no matter what we have experienced in life and no matter what is happening around us, we can still live in a state of health and resilience. Being resilient doesn't mean that we will never get sick or encounter difficulties in life, but it is all about how we relate to the challenges life brings to us and having the right understanding and awareness. Let us embrace whatever comes to us with the greatest love and trust that we are all cared for and that life will find its way...

If you need any support on your own healing journey, I would be more than happy to assist you.

Please email me at: aashild.tilrem@gmail.com

About the Author

Åshild Tilrem is an inspirational holistic health coach, critical care nurse, and all around health entrepreneur from Norway. She holds a Master of Science in Health, Nutrition and Environmental studies along with certification in several modalities in the healing arts. She has traveled all around the world in search of the best solutions to regain health and vitality. With her big heart and genuine desire to help people heal and transform, she supports clients in finding their true gifts, recovering from burnout and health challenges, and navigating major life transitions.

Åshild loves to awaken the light within her clients by using a multi-faceted approach to her work. Her strongest gift is to see the larger picture and help people connect the dots and bring them back to health and wholeness.

Learn more about Åshild here: www.ashildtilrem.com

Contact Åshild via email: aashild.tilrem@gmail.com

STRESS AWARENESS

Are you aware of the things that cause you stress? Becoming aware of your stress triggers will help you be more aware of when you're reactions may get out of hand. And you can then prevent disaster by having an alternative in mind. What are your stress triggers?

Think of the last time you felt annoyed, edgy or irritable. Make a list of the things you know will set you off. For example, when I am forced to wait for people I become irritated and can easily lose my cool.

Now write down at least 3 ways to avoid or prevent those stressful things from happening.

_____

_____

_____

Example:

When I have too many tasks to complete I can become stressed and anxious.

Solutions:

1. Create a time management plan that outlines the time needed to complete each task. And do not overbook

or over commit yourself to more tasks than fit into your daily routine.

2. Do the boring or least fun tasks first to get them out of the way. Having too many burdensome tasks on your to-do list can drain energy and perpetuate stress.

3. Plan to have short breaks in your day to give yourself a positive boost. A quick walk, listening to good music or reading a joke-a-day book can provide relief from monotonous tasks and the sense of overwhelm.

Since part of what makes us feel stressed is the false belief that we are not capable of dealing with the situation, it is best to proactively prepare a few coping mechanisms so that you feel ready to face the challenge. Reminding myself of past success or asking for inner guidance helps. What works for you?

Make a list of 3-5 things you'll do when you are faced with the next stressful situation.

_____

_____

_____

_____

_____

Make time for self-care

The most resilient people ensure that they take care of themselves by addressing stress and other emotions before they get out of control. Highly resilient people who are deeply committed to a life of service recognize that compassion fatigue and burnout can be avoided if they take care of themselves, establish clear boundaries and make fun or lighthearted activities a regular part of their lifestyle. Here are more insightful ways to care for yourself.

Stimulants, chill-pills and sleep

Each of us reacts to sleep deprivation, dietary restrictions, uppers and downers in different ways. So respecting your human engine should also be part of your resilience regimen.

As it pertains to your fuel and energy sources, be mindful of how your body reacts to the amount of sleep you get each night. Most nights it is ideal to get between 7 and 9 hours. I have rarely been able to sleep more than 8 hours and I function like an energized bunny. That's just my nature. I rebound quickly after periods of stress and extreme activity. In fact, I never needed stimulants or caffeine until I went to medical school where I finally developed an affinity for coffee — but it always took lots of milk, sugar and vanilla powder to make it palatable. When I changed to a vegan plant-based lifestyle I stopped drinking coffee altogether. I don't like feeling dependent on a substance and hated the withdrawal headaches. (read on for my new energy boosting routine.)

Whether you drink a lot of coffee or caffeinated beverages, also take into account how easily you can relax and calm down. Do you use alcohol or some sort of downer to unwind? While many claim the health benefits of coffee and red wine, it's helpful to be honest about the downside of using them to rev up or wind down. Is the potential for abuse, dependence or addiction worth it?

Consider using natural products to provide your energy boost when needed. I've replaced coffee with my daily cocktail of matcha, maca root, guarana powder mixed with turmeric and vitamin C salts. I've also decided to take a personalized formula of amino acid supplements which are known to promote vitality, reduce inflammation and boost energy. The antioxidant, mental concentration and immune boosting properties of this new daily regimen keeps me going and helps my body rebound from stressful periods.

Release, refuel, refocus

How do you release the stress and tension you experience every day? Letting go of the pressure to perform and deliver should be a regular part of your day to day existence. Just because we can take on the problems of the world doesn't mean we should. At least not all of the time.

My mother released stress through gardening, while reading her historical romance novels, and reveling in the pleasures of human life — such as ice cream, chocolate and dancing. She got recharged by letting go of work when she handed over the patient list to her colleagues, not taking by taking it home and ruminating over it constantly.

I actually release stress through vigorous exercise. I love brisk walking with hip-hop music in my ears and when I personally experienced the mind-body benefits of hot yoga last year, I became a new fan. Exercise not only gives me a brain boost of feel-good endorphins, it also allows me to leave the stress of the day behind me.

When we allow ourselves the space and time to release the worries, tension and stress of our day we can refocus on what really matters. It is in the times that I've let go of the need to do, do and do that I have had epiphanies about how many things I've said yes to that were not even in alignment with my values and vision for my life! And this awareness allows us to take a bold step toward reclaiming our time, power and our voice to express what we really want in life and what we will no longer tolerate. It also prevents us from using and abusing food, drugs, sex, alcohol or mindless TV watching and Internet surfing to numb ourselves.

Self-care is not selfish

Self-care is about self-preservation

Self-care is not a luxury, it's a necessity

Make a commitment to prioritize the activities that allow you to release tension, recharge your batteries and refocus on the way you really want to live your life. Whether through meditation, yoga, walking, gardening, journaling or pampering with massage or spa treatments, you owe it to yourself. And while you get used to making yourself a priority, bear in mind that caring for yourself will allow you to care even more deeply and genuinely for those you love.

I'm grateful for the example I had in my fierce and feisty mother. She modeled for me the benefits and healthy normality of caring for, honoring and nurturing oneself, which allows us to be fully present and truly of benefit to those we care about. I'm certain that the way she personalized her own self-care routine allowed her to maintain her health and vitality in defiance of her genes, which enabled her to avoid Alzheimer's dementia for nearly 20 years longer than any of her siblings[1].

---

[1] Explore how living a resilient lifestyle helped me and my mother cope with dementia by visiting www.andreapennington.com/category/caring-for-mom/

Resilience Trait #2
Flexibility & Adaptability

In the last chapter, we looked at the number one trait of highly resilient people — Insight. Having the self-awareness to recognize our own triggers empowers us to avoid the situations that will cause us undue stress, or at least to be better prepared for them.

Throughout the ages, wise people have been aware of the traits of resilience. Two and a half centuries ago, Socrates' only teaching was to 'know thyself', but Socrates also demonstrated the importance of the number two trait of highly resilient people — Flexibility.

In Plato's *Republic* (380 BC), we find Socrates getting stuck into deep discussions about what makes a good person, different types of government and the qualities of leadership. Time and again, as those around him try to answer these questions with carefully worded definitions, Socrates uses his own distinctive process of questioning to reveal the flaws in their arguments. At every turn, they are forced to recognize that what might be true in one circumstance cannot be generalized to all other possible scenarios. Every situation is different, and we need to be flexible in our approach.

Socrates' determination to seek truth rather than settling for a black and white perspective of the world eventually led to his death. We are hardwired to generalize and to create default rules of thumb that we can apply to situations without too much thought. This is a great mechanism for allowing us to make quick decisions and conserve mental energy for more demanding tasks. Unfortunately, however, it can also lead to a rigid mindset that prevents us from seeing situations from other perspectives.

The more fixed our mindset is, the more we will struggle to cope with aspects of reality that we can neither accept nor change, and this leads to increased stress and eventually the possibility of burnout. We have to learn to strike a balance between our expectations of how the world should be and the way it is at any given moment. We can't force any person or situation to change to suit our needs, but we can change to adapt to our world.

Philosopher, and theologian, Reinhold Niebuhr captures this spirit of flexibility in his famous 'Serenity prayer':

'God, grant me the serenity to accept the things I cannot change, the courage to change the things I can, and the wisdom to know the difference.'

Accepting the things that we cannot change is the key to dealing with the challenges that life throws at us. It stops us falling into the trap of crying over spilt milk and allows us to focus our mental energy on seeking the best outcome for any given situation — adaptability. Acceptance leads to flexibility. Being flexible is the first step to figuring out how to deal with adversity.

The Taoist teaching of impermanence also steers us away from becoming attached to fixed ideas. Paradoxically, according to Taoism, the only certainty is change. This concept is captured in the Taoist symbol, the taijitu or 'yin-yang' sign, which illustrates the constant interplay between light and dark. The presence of a small white circle in the black half of the symbol and a small black circle in the white half shows how the universe is in a constant state of flux between absolutes. We don't live in a black and white world. Reality is a constantly changing shade of grey, and the more we embrace it just as it is right now, the easier it is to adapt to it.

According to research carried out by Mohammed Al-Mosalwi and Tom Johnson and reported in their paper, In an Absolute State: Elevated Use of Absolutist Words Is a Marker Specific to Anxiety, Depression, and Suicidal Ideation (Clinical Psychological Science, January 2018), depressed people are significantly more likely to use 'absolutist' words such as 'always', 'nothing' and 'completely'. These words reflect a more fixed, rigid perspective on life, don't they? They suggest a world where everything follows a plan, but life's not like that. When was the last time life pitched you a curve ball?

Another notable finding from the Al-Mosalwi and Johnson study is that depressed people are more likely to use first-person pronouns such as 'me', 'myself' and 'I', which suggests that they are more self-preoccupied than people in general. If we only ever consider ourselves in any situation — focusing on how we feel about things, how we think the world should be, and what we want to happen —we become more entrenched in our own single-minded perspective. That makes us less flexible, which in turn will mean we are more unwilling to adapt and less capable of it.

Remember, truth can look different depending on our perspective. What can look like number nine to one person could be a six to another. Paying attention to others, finding out how others see the world, broadens our own perspective and makes us more open minded. Looking at things from more than one perspective is one of the magic ingredients of creativity, which is one of the keys to adaptability.

Being adaptable makes us more agile and better able to adjust our plans to meet changes in the world around us. Sometimes, the most unlikely plan is the one that gets us where we need to be. Sometimes, it's the plan that seems to break all the rules that delivers the best outcome. Thinking creatively lets us consider more options.

Our next personal story, this time relating to the importance of being flexible and adaptable, is written by a man who started out as a performing artist on Broadway. Bruce Cryer is a true Renaissance man who has been thriving into a diverse range of careers since his days in musical theatre. He shows us how being flexible not only enabled him to overcome life-threatening illnesses but to be able to adapt and thrive, making a full recovery while discovering things about himself along the way.

In Bruce's opinion, there are four key elements of human resilience — physical, emotional, mental and spiritual — and these all need to be nurtured equally for all-round health and wellbeing. That means we have to be flexible physically, emotionally, mentally and spiritually.

Bruce also talks about the importance of creativity as a factor of resilience. He believes that everyone is creative, even if they are not artistic, and he shares techniques we can all practice to reconnect with our own creativity.

Our next author, Eric Gerson, is almost the perfect embodiment of flexibility and adaptability. His rock-solid faith in himself, complete refusal to dwell on the past or the future, and strong awareness of what his heart was telling him, allowed him to embrace a lifestyle that many would consider foolhardy.

Eric's story is a prime example of having the wisdom to know when to accept things we can't change and when to change the things we can. His life has been no bed of roses, but as he puts it, he never saw challenges as things to be overcome or mountains to be climbed — they were cones to be navigated around.

Resilience 2.0 – Dawn of the Renaissance Human
by Bruce Cryer

The doctor gets right to the point. "All the tests confirm you have a large tumor, and it's definitely *cancer*."

That word you never want to hear.

Ever.

A word with more emotional baggage than just about any other word in the English language.

I sit there, staring down a dark tunnel and wondering where the heck I'm going. It's not a pretty feeling.

I'll save the details of my two-year healing journey for later in this chapter, but the good news is that, ten years later, I'm cancer-free, and everything else that was damaged or needed repair is working great and much better than expected.

I'm even getting younger, in body, mind and spirit.

My story has a "happy ending" especially due to the dedication I had for many years, prior to my first diagnosis, to developing my own *resilience*.

Lucky me. Very lucky me.

In 1980 I became friends with a visionary named Doc Childre. Ten years later he founded the Institute of HeartMath, which would become acclaimed as one of the most innovative research organizations in the world exploring stress, human performance, heart-brain interactions, and resilience.

Before HeartMath Doc invited me to be part of the founding team as well as the core leadership team. I was deeply involved in developing the HeartMath system that would be expressed through books, workshops, seminars, train the trainer programs, and personal biofeedback technology.

As HeartMath's research grew, it became clear that stress and resilience were two sides of the same coin. As stress occurs in the body, you draw on your reserves of resilience to counteract it. The more resilience you have, the more defense you have against stress. However, the less resilience you have, the more susceptible you are to letting stressful events drain and deplete your energy. Chronic stress provides a constant drain on your resilience, and diet and exercise just aren't enough to get it all back.

The Four Elements of Human Resilience

As we studied hundreds and eventually thousands of individuals across the world, one of the things that became clear was that there are *four dimensions of human energy*, that are all connected and integrated, and are directly related to how much resilience we have in our system.

It's All Connected

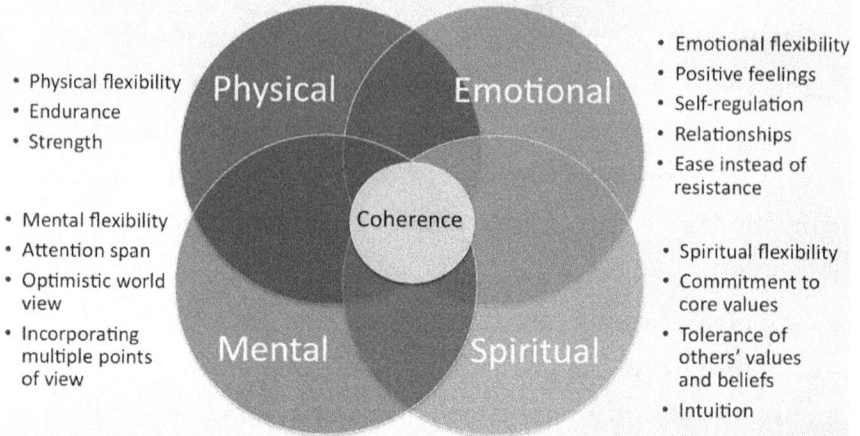

- Physical flexibility
- Endurance
- Strength

Physical

Emotional

- Emotional flexibility
- Positive feelings
- Self-regulation
- Relationships
- Ease instead of resistance

Coherence

- Mental flexibility
- Attention span
- Optimistic world view
- Incorporating multiple points of view

Mental

Spiritual

- Spiritual flexibility
- Commitment to core values
- Tolerance of others' values and beliefs
- Intuition

Copyright 2019 HeartMath Institute

None of these dimensions exists in isolation. Physical trauma can leave massive mental and emotional consequences. Chronic emotional stress, anxiety or fear can affect our physical body in severe ways, even resulting in chronic illness. Mental preoccupations or brain fog can cause accidents or distraction or performance lapses, affecting safety, effectiveness and other unsavory outcomes. Spiritual questioning or depression can deplete our energy and affect all of the other dimensions.

However, balance, integration and positivity within these dimensions can bring tremendous fulfillment, energy, youthfulness, and... Resilience.

This is what I learned, first-hand. If these dimensions are out of balance, some level of dysfunction will occur in one or more of these integrated dimensions, *affecting all the others*. It's physics. It can't *not* happen.

Fortunately, when our resilience is high and that extra "tank" of energy is available to us when life reveals an unexpected challenge or trauma, we may still be deeply affected (we're human after all!) but we can bounce back more quickly than if our resilience was low.

When we're effectively managing stress and building resilience, here's what else is happening: our *insight increases*, we can *bounce back from adversity*, *adapt*, be *flexible*, *persist* in the face of daunting problems, find *tolerance* and *compassion*, be *confident* and *optimistic* when others would doubt or worry, stay *connected* to others instead of isolating ourselves, and experience *positive emotions* and find *meaning* in life.

If you wanted to cook up a huge batch of resilience and be able to sip on it every day of your life, the ingredients for the recipe of that fantastic elixir would be all those words in italics above.

Those are the Top Ten Traits of Resilience. They are truly *synergistic*: activating any of them fortifies and multiplies the power of the others. I believe these traits are key to developing resilience, both in my 25+ years of work as part of HeartMath, and as a cancer survivor, staph infection (MRSA) survivor, double hip replacement thriver, salmonella poisoning survivor and one or two other dramatic-sounding adventures I endured.

Resilience was key to my recovery. Resilience, fueled by the ten traits, was the energy cell I relied upon. I had no idea, even with all the years of developing and teaching the HeartMath system, let alone in practicing the stress-reducing, resilience-enhancing HeartMath techniques, that I would ever need resilience as much as I did during those two years, a period that also included the passing of my mother, and the ending of my marriage.

Okay everybody, *breathe*. Relax. I made it through. With flying colors. I'm healthy now, vibrant, and extremely grateful.

Grateful for the support of so many friends, family and health professionals during that dark period, and …

Grateful that the human system contains the capacity for enormous healing. Resilience is key.

What I learned

The period of 2009-11 and the next few years were a rollercoaster of emotions, physical symptoms, diagnoses, procedures and surgeries, treatments, and waiting.

Waiting to hear results. Waiting to get stronger. Waiting for life to feel hopeful again. Waiting to gain clarity on what all this meant for the next phase of my life.

Gradually a light appeared at the end of the dark tunnel as treatments succeeded and the cancer disappeared. So did the staph infections. While it took months of physical therapy and personal training to regain flexibility and strength in my hips and legs, eventually it did come back. To my amazement, delight, and eternal gratitude.

I never imagined or even hoped I would be able to dance again, but dancing I am. Now powered by two titanium hips!

Better than expected

One of the aspects that stood out during my healing process was the number of times a doctor, a nurse, a friend or family member would see me after a procedure or hospital stay, and say something like "You're looking much better than I expected." This backhanded compliment was followed by me saying, "Well how bad did you think I was going to look?"

But humor aside, I began to realize that my own resilience, hard-won through many years of practicing HeartMath's stress-reducing techniques, had indeed built a deep cellular reservoir of resilience that was never fully depleted. This resilience was available to me to heal and then to thrive, and then to have a personal renaissance in the rediscovery of my innate creativity. I made sure to cultivate and replenish it every day in ways I'll describe shortly.

In fact, the healing period was lightened and energized considerably by an ever-growing desire to *express myself creatively again*. Whether it was taking pictures of the morning dew while an IV bag dripped strong antibiotics into my arm, or sitting in the sunshine in between tentative walking trips on my new hips, I could feel a new energy being born inside myself.

Deep in my bones, in my heart, soul, *everywhere,* I knew I needed to create again. I wanted to sing, to dance, to take photographs, to curate events where I could perform with others and inspire audiences to realize that recovery and a personal renaissance are indeed possible.

Resilience to creativity

In my work as a corporate executive, mentor, and creativity coach, I have come to realize that *everyone is innately creative.* This capacity is programmed into our DNA. The fact that *every human being has the power to create life itself* means the *power of creation is alive inside of us all along.*

Some of us are fortunate to have been raised in home or educational environments that encouraged creative expression and innovative thinking. But most of us were not. Some of us discovered certain artistic skills early in life and felt comfortable thinking of ourselves as creative, but most did not.

Let me make a bold statement: **every human being is designed to create life. Therefore all human beings are fundamentally creative.**

Creating a life is the ultimate act of human creativity which springs from the creative life force present in everyone.

Unfortunately, the vast majority of Earth's inhabitants are only using a fraction of their creative capacity. There's massive opportunity for growth.

Your own renaissance

I see the human journey as a series of births throughout life. Some are biological, like puberty and menopause; others are psychological resulting from education, career choices or travel. Whatever the "cause", new talents and skills are born and strengthened in us based on life events and opportunities.

My recovery from the two year health ordeal became a *renaissance,* a rebirth not only of my physical health and well-being, but of my creative nature as well.

I believe all people are Renaissance Humans, each on our own unique journey through life where we get to birth new parts of ourselves as much as we want.

Let me say it again: we are all fundamentally creative.

Some people may be more *artistic* than others, but that doesn't mean they are more *creative.* Artistic expression is merely one aspect of creative.

Think about the school teacher who can manage unruly kids and energize their learning. They are every bit as creative as the artist or the poet. Consider the customer service representative who calms an upset customer and turns them into a loyal advocate for the company. Imagine the first responder who enters a scene of tremendous chaos to save a life and restore order and humanity. These are all examples of *creativity in action.*

I have discovered several steps that anyone in any phase of life can take to regain, or develop for the first time, their innate creativity. These steps are based on my own journey back to a creative, resilient life; a process that unfolded intuitively.

I especially want to acknowledge Stanford University's Healthy Living Program, which is a central part of Stanford's comprehensive wellness and well-being program for staff and faculty of the University. I have been teaching the HeartMath program there in various formats and departments since 1997. In early 2017, Wes Alles, Ph.D., director of the program and an acclaimed researcher in Type A behavior and employee wellness, commissioned me to create a new multi-session course based on what I had learned in my recovery from resilience to creativity.

Wes's team fast-tracked the launch of the course which we call: **Creativity as Your Personal Well-Being Strategy**.

The program is based on my **Five Catalysts to Awaken Creativity:**
- Mindfulness (with heart)
- Movement
- Nature
- Playfulness
- Artistic Expression

Being creative in extreme or tense situations can be very challenging, but I have learned in my own process, and in working with dozens of executives and managers, these five principles can get us in the right "flow" to come up with new ideas we might have never dreamed were possible. There is also abundant research, which I cite in my course, that being in a creative flow of any kind – writing, singing, dancing, painting, gardening, literally anything that involves creative input – generates positive emotions which biochemically alter our physiology and are the underpinning of new levels of resilience.

In addition, the mental and emotional well-being that happens from doing creative things boosts our attitudes and broadens our perspectives, so the problems we had before the creative activity diminish in intensity, trimmed down to *mole hill* size instead of *mountain*.

Resilience fuels creativity, which builds new resilience, which leads to more energy to create and enjoy life.

Pretty neat formula.

Mindfulness

From the point of view of the Five Catalysts, it begins with being more mindful every day of the thoughts and feelings that block our creative thinking and actions. Things like, "I'm just not a creative type; I'm more of a numbers guy." Or, "I'm too busy to be creative. I've got to get the job done." Or, "I don't have time to waste so all this creativity gibberish sounds so elementary school."

Those thoughts and others block the creative flow that is required to be more effective in our work *and* in our relationships. Mindfulness especially allows us to be fully aware of subtle signals inside and around us that could lead to creative breakthroughs.

Movement

A significant discovery I had was that many a creative block is dislodged by *simply moving*. (When you're healing from hip replacement surgery you become keenly appreciative of what movements you are able to do and which are prevented until healing occurs. As progress and healing happen, the sense of youthful exhilaration is profound!)

Let's remember that many of us lead lives spent sitting for hours and hours on end in front of computer monitors or smartphones. We rarely move. Creativity is energy in action. Creativity is a flow of ideas that results in a new product, a new plan, a poem, a song, a dance…wherever the creative flow is designed to go.

If you're going to sit there like a data zombie all day, don't be shocked when creative ideas don't come running your way. Get up and frickin' move! (This is shockingly effective.)

Dance is my favorite form of movement. Give me some music and I'll make a dance. But when dancing through Times Square seems a little too "made for TV", brisk walking will do just fine.

What's your favorite way to move?

Nature

Nature is well-known to be the muse of many an artist, poet, musician, photographer, and even inventor. It is also the source of some of our greatest refreshment -- like when we take a walk on the beach to "clear our head" so we can make a tough decision. Or when we go out into the sunshine after too many hours and too many days indoors.

Nature helps clear our mind and allows us to feel again the natural rhythms and forces beyond ourselves. This is key to finding our creative flow. Be like nature. Flowing, changing, creating.

There is also a sublime, magnificent and awe-inspiring beauty to nature that refreshes our cellular vitality and builds resilience in and of itself. Yet many of us have become habituated and even numb to the Nature we find near our homes and fail to fully appreciate its restorative, resilience-building effects. Especially in the dark cold months of winter, or the endless days of rain in some parts of the world, our relationship with Nature can feel unfriendly. Do you ever blame Nature for your mood?

When you think about it, how much energy do you spend, and therefore waste, complaining because Nature – in the form of weather – isn't acting to suit your preference. What a waste of energy this is! A guaranteed resilience-depleting process. Stop it, please. (I've done it by the way, many times, especially in the last 18 months after leaving the moderate pleasant sunny climate of my California home of more than 30 years for the much harsher climate of New York.)

Playfulness

During my health journey I realized how important it is to find a playful attitude. There were plenty of reasons to be worried, fearful, anxious, angry, or even despondent. Yet my own knowledge of physiology and emotion taught me that if I had any chance to make a full recovery it would not result from non stop complaining and worrying. I needed to adopt a more light-hearted approach.

Growing up with a very playful mother, as well as fun-loving brothers and relatives made it much easier. Granted I had some hardened patterns of worry and anxiety that needed softening, but playfulness was the perfect elixir.

Playfulness comes naturally to kids. We've all seen kids creating worlds out of their imagination into the sand castles on the beach, or into the action heroes they're scripting, or the puppets that come alive in their hands. The energy of playfulness takes the density out of situations, a heaviness and gravity that feels like lead weights around our ankles when our imagination wants to soar.

Artistic expression

The fifth catalyst, Artistic Expression, is where the rubber meets the road.

Trying new forms of Artistic Expression activates our brain to build new circuitry, circuitry that will come in handy when any creative need arises. Our brain is literally creating new neural circuits every time we try anything new, and when it's a creative activity multiple resources within the brain are marshaled to create the solution.

I have watched people who had convinced themselves "I'm not creative" and then they discover an authenticity in their soul when they write, or discover a child-like freedom when they dance, or express deep feelings through a photographic essay or poem, or experience a connection to the Earth and to some primal energy when they throw pottery or create sculpture.

You don't have to do all five Catalysts every day to lead a creative, resilient life. But the regular practice of each of them can provide stepping stones to awaken your Creative Brilliance once and for all.

You, the Renaissance Human, are awakened.

What's Next?

Here are some tips for how to use what I've shared.

1. Explore where you're "wasting" energy worrying over things you can't change.
2. Put more "heart" in your life and your work through more compassion, more gratitude, more love, and especially more self-care.
3. Get up and move when you've been sitting too long or feeling blocked creatively.
4. Get out in Nature and appreciate its magnificence. Breathe in the vitality. Feel warmed and relaxed by the sunshine, a cool breeze, a walk by the ocean or a river.
5. Find ways to take life less seriously and become more playful.
6. Try poetry, or creative writing, or salsa dancing, or a photography or art class, or crafts or gardening.
7. Expand your comfort zone to live life more fully, with less fear, less anxiety, and more fun.
8. Repeat as needed, ☺ as often as possible.

About the Author

Bruce Cryer has had a diverse career spanning musical theater, biotech, personal development, health and well-being, and executive coaching. He began as a singer/dancer/actor on Broadway, including two years in *The Fantasticks*, the world's longest running musical. Since the early 90s, Bruce has brought the HeartMath program optimal health, business success, personal balance, and human performance to organizations such as Stanford Business School, Mayo Clinic, Kaiser, NASA, Unilever, Shell, and the NHS.

Bruce is co-author of *From Chaos to Coherence: The Power to Change Performance* and the *Harvard Business Review* article "Pull the Plug on Stress". Since 1997 Bruce has been adjunct faculty at Stanford.

A two year health crisis convinced him to focus his energies on healing and creativity. He recently released *Renaissance Human,* an album of original songs co-created with the Brothers Koren.

Bruce mentors visionary entrepreneurs, gives keynote *performances* and teaches on the connection between Creativity and Well-Being at venues around the world.

Visit Bruce online at www.RenaissanceHuman.com

What's Ebay?
by Eric Gerson

"What's Ebay?"

I often wonder had I known the profound consequences that question would have on my life, if I would still have mustered the courage to ask. After hearing a coworker explain to a friend that they had to pack some dishes they sold on the site, I inquired and was instantly hooked.

Within 2 weeks and after borrowing some cash from Mom and Dad to buy one of those oversized vintage computers, I was on my journey. This would mark the end of the last "real job" I would ever hold. Since then, I have held daily gratitude for having the guts to ask, "What's Ebay?", and for developing perfect faith in myself to follow the trail it would lead me down over the next 20+ years.

Living on the little strip of land known as Virginia's Eastern Shore, merchandise ripe for resale was abundant. Traipsing around in my beat-up old sedan, sometimes with my wife and infant son in tow, weekends were spent at yard sales, thrift stores and auctions.

"This is EASY", or so I thought. You see, it was 1999, or what online sellers now refer to as "back in the day". Essentially, anything I listed was such a rare find that it sold like hotcakes. The selling process was easy, fees were cheap, and online shopping was the new time saving trend everyone was eager to try. Profit margins were so ridiculous it would have been easy to get sucked into thinking I would soon be a millionaire if I could just get enough capital. Little did I know that while laying the foundation for my business had felt charmed, challenges would follow to test my resolve.

A few months after asking the question, "What's Ebay?", I had a new business and found myself back in Florida. My now ex-wife was a bit of a gypsy, and though it would taste a lie to blame it all on her, the 15 moves in the first 20 years of marriage was the drumbeat to my life as a self-employed stay at home Dad. The thousands of constant changes that came were met with the same resolve and courage I would employ whenever presented with a challenge. I had a firm belief in myself and in my abilities, something others might mistake for arrogance. But most importantly I lacked the ability to look forward in fear or back with regret. Regardless of outcome I never questioned any of my decisions. I just used whatever result came as a stepping stone and kept moving forward. So, when life brought me back to Florida, the choice between a real job and selling online presented itself, but I held firm and steady in the face of enormous pressure from friends and family who felt I should do the responsible thing by working for someone else.

The next two years brought endless opportunities to reinvent myself, highlighted by the birth of my daughter and followed by my son's Autism diagnosis. Life became a whirlwind of doctor appointments, online medical research and keeping the oddest work hours ever invented. Still, the economic atmosphere translated into easy sales and flowing money. Oh, not enough to be considered rich, but just enough to spend too much eating out and at theme parks. It still seemed as though things were easy for me, but hindsight has taught me that it was my faith in myself that created that illusion. When you do not question yourself, results are easily painted as positive. So even with the hecticness of a newborn and a disabled child, I felt secure in my own shadow. I did not view those things as adversity to be overcome, but rather as traffic cones to navigate while staying on the same road. Then, on Sept 11, 2001, the ease with which things had come to me vanished by days end.

So far, I had sailed through the seas of family and business rather smoothly, so while it took courage and faith to follow the unconventional path I had chosen, things were good, and outside pressures were at a minimum. The events of 9/11 changed all that. Obviously, sales stopped, as in almost zero, for the next 7-10 days. Proper planning had allowed me the luxury of enough back-stock, so buying new merchandise was not an immediate issue. Still, by the time things normalized, monthly income was cut in half for the next 18 months. With my family accustomed to a certain "Disney" lifestyle, the pressure mounted that maybe it was time for another "real" job.

But instead, with a firm belief in myself and confidence in my ability to reinvent myself, I pushed forward, changing and tweaking business models until I found success again. There were some lean times, no doubt. There were days I sat waiting for something to sell, so I could pay for dinner that night (Egg sandwiches AGAIN??!!). But here is the catch; something ALWAYS sold. This was my first unintentional experience with the Law of Attraction. I could be broke at 8am but I knew, I just KNEW something would sell so we would have food money for that day. I would go about my day as if the money was there, and without fail, it always was. I am sure from the outside, looking back, it's easy to criticize and maybe even call me negligent in cutting it so close in the care of my family. But that strong and perfect faith in myself allowed me to push worry aside, and act as though the good had already come.

An unquestioning spirit

A few years and a few intrastate moves later I found myself in Palm Bay, Florida, in the home where I would stay the longest, nearly 10 years. Business had settled in nicely, and while it was not the heyday of pre 9/11, we were living more month to month than minute to minute. Still, the daily challenges were abundant, and the strain on my marriage was showing. While I remained constant in my stay at home status, my wife flirted with a career, taking and leaving several jobs, then coming back home to work with me until her internal pressure cooker went off again. This left me in a constant state of reinvention, not only of the business, but of myself.

The challenge of raising an Autistic child was enormous enough, however doing so while managing a home-based business, in addition to my partner's unstable work situation proved daunting. Monthly changes to "how things are done" became the norm, whether it was who would do the grocery shopping or who was listing items for sale, it was quite literally constant change. This again is where an unquestioning spirit comes into play. To be successful in such an atmosphere, you must be able to make a quick decision and accept the outcome as another opportunity, rather than a consequence. Nothing is good or bad, it just is. If one product no longer sells, find another. Eventually, the old product will sell again and now you have two good products rather than one. Taking what others would interpret as a negative and finding a way to turn it into a positive is probably my greatest attribute, and is a trait you must possess to be a success in whatever path you choose.

As life would have it, once things settled into a nice comfortable routine, it was shockingly blown up. Despite having a tubal ligation when giving birth to our daughter, my wife became pregnant with our second son! While she struggled with acceptance, I reveled in the fact that spirit had told me 6 weeks prior that she was with child. Little did I know this would eventually lead me to my create another business model in which I would employ the same principles. But back then, my attitude about the pregnancy was one of laughter (not appreciated by the way) around the idea that we HAD some things planned out that would no longer be possible, and I am pretty sure this was the last time I allowed for planning that went past the "what's for dinner" stage. In yet another unexpected turn he would be born Autistic as well, bordering on the edge of what would be considered severe.

So, by 2007 I had two Autistic boys, both in completely different stages while trying to manage what was a declining business model due to a saturation of sellers. Everyone by now knew about online selling, and was trying their hand at it. Armed with an equity loan and a head full of *Storage Wars* type programming, those with "real jobs" were finding out that they could make an extra buck by heading out to auctions and yard sales on the weekends. They were just fine with overspending for product, since they had a paycheck to count on regardless of whether stock sold or not. So, with tons of adversity as the backdrop, I made the quick decision to attempt a slow transition out of online sales and into something more spiritually fulfilling and financially stable, or so I thought.

A transition into failure

Massage school! And why not? I was still relatively young, in good shape, and apparently had "a way" with people. I could fill a novel with the experiences that came out of my massage career, but for now I will simply state the lessons I learned. Regardless of the optics that may show something to be a bad decision, do not let regret manifest fear. Take your lumps and lessons and build success on top of them. Do not allow failure to change the way you make your choices, rather, allow your choices to change the way you look at failure.

In the macro sense, my massage career was a failure for a multitude of reasons, ranging from market saturation to my own failing health. However, had I not stubbornly kept at it , trying a number of times to get it right, I would not be in the space I am today. That experience was the precursor to becoming more aware my intuitive gifts and how to apply them from a Spiritual perspective.

Regardless of outcome, my continued attempts at success, coupled with my current knowledge of WHY I had to learn those lessons, proves to me that the path of least resistance is often disguised as hardships that need to play out. While I am no longer a massage therapist, the lessons learned and pathways that were cleared for me due to failure are currently serving me in ways I could not have dreamed possible, and that far surpasses any success I had hoped for with massage.

by 2009 I found myself in the same position as most, just trying to wrap my head around the financial crisis and how it would affect my business going forward. The next few years can only be described as floating in a pool of accidental good luck. I was nowhere near as focused on any one thing as I should have been, and to be honest, it showed. My online businesses were functional but stagnant. My marriage had begun a rapid decline into the throes of death, although it would take another 10 years of constant reinvention before I would finally release it. My health also took a turn and I experienced weeks where I could not drive due to dizziness, among other symptoms, that I would later find out were the initial stages of Lyme disease.

Shortly after letting go of the fight to keep my marriage alive, the diagnosis and subsequent healing began, a true testament to the Law of Attraction. Letting go is a must. However, knowing when to let go only comes when you have a true direct connection to your own spirit. Once you are ready for the lessons that will move you forward, things will change rapidly and, sometimes violently, so it is important to acknowledge why things are happening, but it is imperative that you do not engage in self blame. Like I said, no looking back with regret. Take each stage of the lesson and build on it.

Looking back over the last 10 years, I feel the need to redefine what most would consider success. Fairy tales teach us to look for happy endings but spirit demands that we acknowledge only happy moments. It's easy to give instruction on how to be successful by trusting one's self and living without fear. But for me, the biggest sign of success is knowing WHEN you have gotten what you asked for, and in recognizing the path you took so you may re-engineer your success over and over again.

Too many times people change course due to the lack of immediate gratification, as we are bombarded daily with messages of how to do things quickly and easily. We are taught to overthink things to the point of paralysis, never knowing if the move we have chosen is the correct one, and we look for those immediate signs to show the way. True success comes in knowing how to play the long game, the macro view rather than micro. Having faith in oneself is only half the battle. It is knowing when to let go that is the tricky part.

The path I started in 1999 has been as bumpy and challenging as one could imagine, yet throughout it all, my internal goal was easily stated. I wanted a simple life, where I could just work a few hours a week and have the rest of the time to enjoy nature, spend time with my dogs and live in a rural environment near water. I simply lived as though I knew those things would happen, without focusing on HOW they would manifest. Despite multiple attempts and failures, they taught me lessons that led to my eventual success.

Today is Tuesday, an early summer afternoon. I just got back from the river about a quarter mile from my home where I take my 3 dogs for a swim almost daily. My house smells like wet dog and the furniture looks like a sheep slept on it. I am located in an area that is more perfectly what I would have wanted than anything I could imagine. I now work, maybe 15 hours a week, unless it's the Holiday season, and I support my family just fine, with plenty of extra time left over for the very things I set out to enjoy 20 years ago. If someone were to ask me how, the answer would not be what they expect. It's not about being good at business or working late into the night. It's not even about that $600 my parents loaned me for my first computer. The answer is simple. A perfect faith in myself. The simple knowledge that by following my own heart and spirit without fail, I would reach my goal, so long as I did not allow the multitude of failures and recalculations to deter me from my path. It sounds so easy, and in many ways it can be.

My new life partner has a saying, "Nothing changes until something changes" and I would add that "Everything changes when something changes." As life would have it, things have changed for me once again career wise. While my online business still exists, Karan and I have started a new endeavor that brings people the support they need when dealing with their own life challenges. Through my clairvoyance & intuition, and Karan's experience in working with hospice families, both in nursing and support roles, we have combined our strengths to form a unique duo. While I get messages from my spirit, or the spirits of others, Karan has a gift in explaining the messages and flowing the conversation to allow for clients to have a clear understanding of how the messages relate to their current challenge. The transition to this new business has been one of the most difficult challenges of my life, however applying the same perfect faith that I used all those years ago has eased that some, and has reminded me of the most important lesson I have learned.

Trust yourself, follow your own advice, and in the instances where you turn out wrong, learn from it so that you do not repeat the same mistakes twice. A life of abundance awaits us all, provided we are ready, and unafraid to claim it.

About the Author

Eric's innate belief and practice of Law of Attraction enabled him to manifest the business, life partner, and lifestyle he visioned. Perfect faith and unrelenting resilience is his secret. In addition to his home-based business, Eric is a storyteller and enjoys creative endeavors that bring others laughter and a little irreverent humor! With his life partner, Karan Joy Almond, he runs a consulting business for people who feel ready to approach their life challenges in a wholistic manner.

Eric can hear, feel, and sense beyond the five senses to help clients figure out where they are stuck. Karan uses her medical background with Astrology and Human Design elements to help clients use the information Eric gets. Together, they have both overcome personal illness and life traumas that have prepared them for the work they do together. Both have an affinity for end of life clients and caregivers.

Please visit www.themanifestingmedium.com for more information on contacting Eric and Karan. Check out their book, *How To Survive the 2020 Election by Living a Law of Attraction Life.*

Resilience Trait #3
Persistence

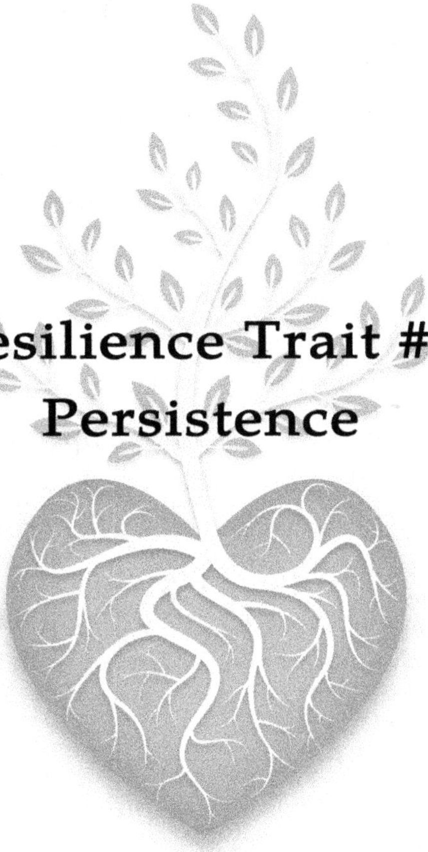

Persistence is an essential quality for resilience that can be cultivated by anybody, regardless of your situation, experiences or current approach to life's challenges. It does not mean the dogged pursuit of accolades or approval from others, but rather the inner quality of determination that means you keep putting one step in front of the other, even when times get tough.

The most resilient people have incredible tenacity. They believe in the exponential power of small steps and no matter how they feel, they find the energy, willpower and courage to keep on taking them. Even when the outcome is not guaranteed and the destination is uncertain, having persistence is a key trait when it comes to not letting your circumstances dictate your destiny.

Without persistence you will give up too easily, let the opinions of others dictate your direction and let circumstances weigh you down. A lack of persistence can mean you stay stuck, you feel powerless and you lack any sense of vitality. Far better to find a way to take the smallest step forward, so that you start aligning with your best self again.

Persistence can often be perceived negatively, as there are times when it is driven by the pursuit of an outcome that is more about proving yourself and satisfying your ego. This type of persistence tends to be exhausting to maintain and it has little to do with resilience.

Scientists studying resilience have found that those who keep working towards overcoming their situation by maintaining constant focus and effort, are the ones who emerge most successfully from whatever it is they are dealing with. This is true whether the situation is a scary diagnosis, a mental health issue, loss of a loved one or any number of other life transitions. The motivating factor is generally stronger than any sense of fear that arises when looking at the big picture, and momentum is created by belief in the power of repeated small steps.

To do this requires a strong sense of trust in yourself and in the possibility of a different life. It requires cultivation of the inner belief that you have exactly what it takes to make it through challenging times, even when it feels as though you are trying to walk through treacle. The most resilient people use their challenges as fuel to help them move forwards, which means they become self-reliant when it comes to finding motivation.

Persistent people are motivated not only by the possibility of a more fulfilling future on the other side of their current circumstances, they also delight in the process required to get there — whether they realize it or not. With every small win and every shift forward, they gather more evidence that they have what it takes to shift their reality. This creates a powerful self-fulfilling prophecy, which boosts their confidence and conviction daily, giving them greater staying power.

To develop more persistence, we have to use our insight to identify what lies behind our desire to give up when we are trying to overcome challenges or make changes. Do we give up out of fear, lack of conviction, self-pity or exhaustion? Do we feel as though we are powerless, a victim of circumstances or the only one in the world experiencing this? If these feel true, what contradictory evidence can we gather to boost our belief in our capacity to keep going when the going gets tough?

Our first story is a powerful example of how important it is to examine our inner beliefs, especially when it comes to transforming your future from one of victimhood to powerful creator. Susan Edwards completely rewrote her personal story in her mid thirties, by taking ownership of her circumstances and using them to fuel her as she made up for lost time. Her wounds became her life's work and thanks to persistence, she has subsequently impacted the lives of thousands through her workshops and seminars.

Our next story is from an extremely resilient woman who obstinately refused to give up on herself, despite her life reaching depths that she describes as feeling like a dark cold mist had formed. Berit Bosdal's story transcends continents, spans years and gives us hope that no place is ever too far from home that we cannot find it within us to rise again. Along with persistence, this author also acknowledges curiosity as being a powerful ally on her journey. May your curiosity be awakened as you read her story and may her final recommendations help you to strengthen your own persistence.

The third story in this chapter illustrates how deeply powerful our connection with our body is when it comes to accessing the inner belief we need to become more resilient. Written by Cynthia Harrison, a soulful woman who had an extremely difficult childhood, this story transcends decades and shows us what it takes to keep going even when you have no support and no one hears or sees you. This author learned to listen deeply to her body and to respect the voice within. These qualities became her strength, even when all she could do was sit in a park and cry.

In our final story in this chapter, Ann Marie Wyrsch paints a very clear picture of what it's like to grow up in a family affected by addiction. Her childhood primed her for a life of missed connections, but she found her way to the 12-step recovery community which helped her make sense of her life. She offers her own 12 step process for the recovering/discovering adult who may have also experienced addiction or codependency.

Persistence to Peace
by Susan Edwards

Over 35 years ago I was emotionally wounded and my inner life was a mess. I looked OK on the outside, but had no inner peace, only devastation on the inside. I decided at that time to be "well." Although I sensed it would take a long time for my hidden wounds to heal, I made an important decision:

"If I am prepared to wait forever, it won't take so long."

In the ensuing years, I never gave up on my Inner Healing Journey and I'm happy to say that I made it! This is my definition of RESILIENCE.

I once read: "I've never met a strong person with an easy past." For me this rings true. My past looked "easy," but was difficult and always hidden. Everything, and I mean everything, looked good on the outside. I was a typical Baby Boomer, living in a Midwestern ranch home, two parents married for 60 years, three healthy children, a comfortable middle class family. Dad, was a bank Vice President, mother a full time homemaker. Brother became a dentist, sister, a dental hygienist. BUT, and this is a big but, I was miserable on the inside for most of my life. Deeply troubled, battling depression, having a wounded cognitive mindset, unsatisfied, and feeling like something was intrinsically wrong with me; something had been omitted; like there was a hole inside of me that was impossible to fill.

Where it all began

When I was one year old, my dad and his two brothers were sent overseas to Europe during WWII. He did not return until I was four years old. During this time my mother lived with her mother-in-Law and two sisters-in-law in the city in one house with three infants born 4 months apart. The three women were not acquaintances before this time, and as the story goes, did not get along.

Periodically, I was told that my mother couldn't take it anymore and took me, the first grandchild, to her parents in the country 50 miles away. Back and forth, back and forth every couple of months.

I have come to believe that the precious baby that my dad knew had disappeared in the three years he was gone. When he returned home at the war's end, what he found instead was a spoiled, bratty, precious child. I later learned that I had been sexually molested by my maternal grandfather, which continued for a number of years. One of the results is that I have very few memories of my dad through most of my life; it was as if he did not exist. I think we were scared of each other. He felt like a stranger.

Because of my strained relationship with my dad, I transferred the father role to God. My picture of God was this: A disapproving, mean, authority figure who was watching and judging me, ready to pounce and back me into a corner from which the one and only escape was to "kill myself". I had been taught and believed suicide was a sin, and I would be condemned to Hell for all eternity. I was trapped!!!! For years in my life as an adult, I would find myself sleep-walking and being awakened by my husband to realize I was in a corner banging on the walls, crying and screaming, "Let me out!! Let me out!!!"

When I was 12 years old, my mother experienced a religious conversion and became a Pentecostal Fundamentalist while my father and his family were Roman Catholics. My father thought all Pentecostals were "crazy" and my mother thought all Catholics were "heathens." From this time on I lived in a home of "Religious Addiction." My parents shuttled us back and forth between churches and fought constantly. Both thought they were trying to keep us from going to Hell. Their fights were verbally and emotionally brutal, not physical, but traumatic for me to witness. It got so horrible that when I was in 7th grade my mother delivered a full-term healthy, 10 pound, beautiful baby boy named Danny, who unexpectedly died in the hospital at three DAYS old! A few weeks later I heard my dad tell my mom that he "was glad the baby died so that she couldn't take it to her church."

I just wanted them to love each other.

Emotional and verbal cruelty were often on display. In my home I always felt like I was wading in thick black sludge, like evil swirling around up to my knees. This began a life filled with dread and a pervading sense of impending DOOM. There was no escape from it.

One Christmas, my mom got a new coat for a present and my dad hated her church so much that he went into her closet and ran chains up through the sleeves and padlocked it to the rod so she couldn't wear it to her church. One Easter as she was leaving for church, he grabbed her darling new pill-box hat off her head and cut off the yellow rose on the top. She was so humiliated. My stomach still turns when I remember this.

I wanted our family to "look good," so I became an over-achiever. I had the 3 "B's" (Beauty, Brains and a Body), and I was even voted as the girl with the prettiest teeth and eyes. I was very popular in High School and very involved in extracurricular activities:

- Cheerleader for 4 years
- Captain of the cheerleading squad for 2 years
- Captain of the volleyball team
- Star guard on the basketball team, I even beat out a senior as Basketball Queen in my junior year.
- President of the National Honor Society, Future Homemakers, and Future Teachers of America
- Played French horn in the band
- Majorette and Baton & Flag Twirler
- Vice-President of the Student Council
- Member of the Girls Athletic Association and, last but not least,
- Salutatorian

My coping strategies

I learned to use males. I used my feminine wiles to get what I wanted. I always dated older guys. My high school steady had already graduated and had a job. He bought a new convertible and I managed to convince him to take the bus to work so I could drive the convertible to school. For me, men were "toys" meant to obey me. Part of my game was to see how far I could push them with the promise of me giving them more, which I never delivered. I have forgiven myself for using them because I know now I was on survival mode and just trying to navigate with the inside turmoil.

In my Senior Year, I remember being miserable. At age 17 I was already burned out. I looked so good on the outside, but inside I looked like raw hamburger. This was going to get worse because I was to become a "Tiny Fish in a Gigantic Pond."

I went away to a large state university where I was overwhelmed. The first day there a photographer spotted me at registration and followed me for three days taking pictures for the Alumni Magazine. It was flattering, but I felt lost and so alone. The first night in the dorm I was invited to a "Purple Passion Party." A party in a cave with a bathtub filled with grape juice and every imaginable type of alcohol. This began a year of drinking. Remember, my mother was a Pentecostal and I had never touched alcohol.

I was really messed up during my Freshman, and only, year in College. I sneaked out of the dorm at night to go drinking. I skipped classes constantly. I did manage to keep my academic scholarship, but I felt lost. I was deeply troubled and unhappy.

I was only at this University for a year, where I met the "man of my dreams." I lost my virginity during this relationship. Because I was raised that this was sinful and shameful, I decided that we had to get married, this was even after he once date raped me in his fraternity house and someone walked in on us. This person did not know that he had torn through my underwear and spread the "news" through his frat house. The shame and humiliation I felt were devastating. But I was addicted to the relationship so we eloped a year later.

I had no idea that I actually picked someone who was more violent than I knew at the time. I found out he had previously been jailed for beating his mother and was involved in an incident on the East Coast with a homosexual being beaten with a chain. I was married for two years and being beaten frequently. I believed he would eventually kill me, but I could not leave.

Finally I was so broken and desperate for a measure of peace that I went to the state mental hospital and saw a psychiatrist when I was 19 years old. I remember that he said: "You will never be well until you establish a relationship with you father." I said: "It will never happen." My dad scared me, not because I was ever physically abused, but for the way he treated my mom. He treated her with contempt and what looked like hatred to me.

But, I did enter intensive psychotherapy for one and a half years and finally got the courage to get a divorce. What I now know is that the main reason for picking such a violent relationship was to manifest how I felt on the inside. I was deeply troubled, depressed, and desperate. I never attempted suicide, but prayed to die constantly.

Finding true love

After the divorce I was not well, but I had survived. It would take many more years of therapy to thrive. I dated many men for the next two years and then I found, Robert Edwards, and fell madly in love. Because by that time I had worked through my early trauma, I picked a kind, loving man who was 14 years older than me. He did fit the profile of a "father image" as he was very handsome, a model and was prematurely gray.

We were very happy for the first three years of our relationship, and then while of vacation he had a major heart attack while water skiing. I was 26 years old. I did not think I could LIVE without a man in my life. I was so angry at him for almost dying. I felt the same abandonment I previously felt with my dad.

He survived and was off work for six months. I went into a dark, deep depression. I did not leave my house for months. I did not bathe for months on end. I lived on cashews and Coca-Cola. Because he was so ill, no one was aware of the horrible condition I was in.

Eventually, months later as he recovered and got well, the depression lifted and three years later we had a daughter. I was diagnosed with postpartum depression two years after her birth and this continued my journey of healing that lasted for decades. I was still determined to get well. Fortunately I had picked the kind of man who stuck with me on the journey. He was kind, loving, faithful and compassionate.

There is no way to adequately synthesize a decades long marriage, but I had found a man who supported, loved and encouraged me through the years. We overcame many struggles and were married for 43 years until his death in 2008. My journey to health required his utmost patience. He supported me through many therapists, bouts of depression, misunderstandings and times of alienation.

During this time his financial support enabled me to build a career with my minuscule formal education. He delighted in my successes and ended up being my best friend. We also had another daughter five years later, who has has given us four precious grandchildren. I am happier today than I have ever been in my entire life. I feel safe.

Healing in community

During my healing journey, I got involved with the Adult Children of Alcoholics Movement (ACofA). It was here that I discovered that even though there may not have been alcohol involved with my dad, the religious addiction had the same effect on me. I totally identified with the others in the program. It was like someone had been living my life, reading my mail. This was the real start of finding answers. I had all of the characteristics and felt like I belonged.

At the beginning of ACofA there were only two books written, but within a relatively short time book store shelves were filled to overflowing.

This was followed by the inner child movement. This also resonated with me and to this day I believe it is a seminal work for emotional, psychological, physical, and psychic health. Thanks to this work, my life took a 180 degree turn. I went from a depressed homemaker always asking: "Is this all there is?" to going back to college and finding my life-long passion.

I took the Miller Analogy Test, a standardized test used for graduate school admissions, then enrolled in a Graduate School Program with only one year of college. I completed an internship entitled "Ministry and Therapy to Adults Raised in Chemically Dependent and/or Dysfunctional Families."

I went on to develop workshops and seminars that I have presented for 35+ years to tens of thousands of people from ages 12 to 90. The subject was "Those Hidden Wounds": Their Effects on our Lives Personally and Professionally." I described the Survival Roles we assume and how to use these roles to serve us and not harm us.

I also was in private practice as a psychotherapist for 30+ years without an undergraduate degree. My healing opened up my world and I have devoted a great part of my life helping hurting adults do the same.

In my presentations, I teach that there are 5 Stages of Healing;

1. Information on the Survival Roles.
2. Insight/Awareness on how to apply the information personally.
3. Behavioral Modification. I call this the Misery Stage where the outside has changed, but the inside is the same.
4. Deep emotional healing. Learning to feel the old feelings, not just talk about them is the hardest part of the journey, because this is where the hidden and old "Pain" is allowed to emerge. It is experiential, not intellectual.
5. Spiritual Maturation/Wholeness. When we have access to our ABC's.
   - Affective: feelings
   - Behavior: acting in our own best interests
   - Cognitive: thinking that is clear, rational

Epilogue

With regard to my parents, I make no blame, judgements or criticism of them. I am over 70 years old now and I believe that they "gave me better than they got," as did my grandparents and great-grandparents before them. When we "know better" we hopefully "do better."

Fortunately I have two adult daughters and because I did my own personal healing work I believe I "gave better than I got." Still, I'm sure I made lots of mistakes, but they were different from the previous generations and I gave them permission to do their own healing work, something I had to do on my own. Over the years, I have forgiven everything, reconciled with my parents and the only thing left is my love and gratitude for the life they gave me.

Healing is a journey and a process. Every step helps us take the next one. I had scores of therapists, counselors, spiritual directors, social workers, psychologists, and psychiatrists, etc., and each one helped me find another piece of the puzzle. Books also have answers. Trust the process. Happiness and emotional health are your birthright.

I wish you joy, hope and peace on your journey,
Susan

About the Author

Susan Edwards, a native of St. Louis, moved to Waco, Texas, eight years after the death of her beloved husband, Robert, to be closer to grandchildren. She holds a Master of Pastoral Studies from Loyola University New Orleans and was a Psychotherapist and Professional Presenter for 35 years.

Her expertise in Family Systems Therapy helps illuminate how the survival strategies we learned in our family of origin affect our lives today. These insights offer hope and a framework to help us approach our challenges and situations more consciously. Over the years, Susan has witnessed "miraculous" changes in her client's lives.

Susan's workshops have been enjoyed by thousands of people of all ages. She is known for her encouraging style and warm sense of humor.

She hopes to travel and present her Workshops to a wider audience and is developing a telephone coaching practice specializing in "Inner Child Healing."

Visit Susan online at www.SusanEdwards.me

When One Door Closes Another One Opens
by Berit Bosdal

As a young girl I was very curious and adventurous. Occasionally that led me to challenge myself beyond my capabilities, and I would find myself unwillingly in the air before crashing down head first, or looking up from under a truck that had to slam on the brakes to avoid running me over. The fact that my family teasingly declared that I had a punching card at the ER never stopped me from pursuing new adventures.

I married young to an adventurous man, we had two children within 18 months, and moved from Norway to live in the exotic land of Japan. From the outside it looked like the perfect fairy tale, but under the surface a dark, cold mist was starting to take form.

It started with postnatal depression triggered by the traumatic delivery of my youngest daughter, complete with post delivery infections, chronic low blood pressure and anaemia. Inch by inch, I was drawn down into a black hole where no light or happiness gets in or out. Feelings like helplessness, isolation and apathy dominated my days.

The marriage ended shortly after with a painful divorce, and I became a part of the modern world's statistics as a single mom. I soon became as busy as a bee working two jobs on top of being a physical therapist at a hospital in

Norway, just to make ends meet. Despair topped with anger became normal feelings for me. The anger gave me energy to push the despair aside so I could function as mom and head of the family, but it also made me exhausted.

Ten years of living in this emotional disharmony knocked me down physically and mentally, and led to a major breakdown. I suffered from chronic fatigue, chronic pain, social anxiety and severe panic attacks. One year of sick leave was not enough to get me back on my feet.

The shift

A career counsellor told me to shift focus and get a master's degree to help me open up to new opportunities. I started laughing. My memory was similar to that of a goldfish, I struggled to stay focused enough to read the newspaper. How on earth would I be able to read a book and remember enough to pass an exam? It sounded like a bad joke. I went home and forgot all about it.

But she had created a spark in me. Through the dark mist in my blurry mind came memories of me enjoying studying and being good at it. Gradually I convinced myself that I could do it again. After all, I wanted to live a different life than the one I was living. I wanted to move away from stress, sickness and fatigue and move towards high energy, good health and strength in my body and mind. There was only one way to do that, and that was to prepare myself to change paths and start walking.

Who better to help me prepare for that walk than my loyal dog Dixie. Together we were training with a Search and Rescue Team, and she became my true companion. Walking and training with her in the forest every day gave me peace in my body and mind. It was like meditation. She reminded me how important connection with animals and nature was for me. Dixie taught me that it is important to have our eyes on the end goal, but more importantly to create secondary aims and celebrate every little bit of success.

With that insight I jumped back into university, eager to feed my mind with knowledge and new experiences.

New opportunities

I had remarried and in the midst of my studies my new husband was asked to work in South Korea for three years. My adventurous soul reignited and I jumped back on the horse and moved to Asia yet again.

Landing in Busan I believed that everything was possible. This was like starting over with a blank sheet of paper and brand new crayons, and I felt my body shiver with joy and anticipation.

My batteries where recharging but I was still not where I wanted to be. Books, mindfulness and exercise had gotten me so far, but I needed more to get further on my path. I had heard about the benefits of meditation but I had never given it a proper chance. What better place to learn meditation than here in Asia?

I was introduced to master Michael and the practice of Kouksundo by a friend. Kouksundo is a traditional mind-body practice that has been used for thousands of years. Master Michael did not speak much English, but was a kind and gentle soul that did his best to communicate on a heart to heart level. Even though I didn't understand the why's of the practice, I fully trusted my master showing me the how's. I left my western medicine education by the front door and trusted the process completely.

Master Michael gently guided me through the routines, but I always felt that there was something I was missing because of the language barrier. I had to learn to listen to my body to gain the knowledge. Gradually I felt stronger, less stressed and more happy.

I completed my masters degree and proved to myself that my brain was back on track and functioning again after years on the back burner. With regained energy and confidence I was ready for a new adventure – working towards a new career.

I asked around and got hired for minor projects at first. This gave me a taste for working with processes in organisational culture and change management. A bigger project gave me the opportunity to help Korean employees increase their engagement and self-efficacy and challenge their culture's status quo. Feeling that I was making a difference and loving it, I was eager for more, but the project ended. The decision maker was not convinced the good results could be duplicated, because in his opinion it had been the most talented that had participated. I was stunned. I knew this wasn't true but still bought into it, but only for a moment.

Obstinate as a mule, I started to read more books and study further on my own. I wanted to learn from my experiences and figure out how I could improve.

I met master Rose after three years of practicing Kouksundo. Under her teachings I understood more of the practise since she was fluent in English. But masters can only give information and guidance — true learning comes through experience. One day as I was doing my breathing technique I felt this sudden ease brushing through every cell of my body. I intuitively knew that this was the feeling of alignment with my true self. Suddenly everything made sense.

Further expansion

The stay in Korea was coming to an end, but I was not ready to move back to Norway. Luckily my husband got a three year contract in London, UK, and I was asked to join a project there. I was over the moon with joy. This would give me more work experience before returning to Norway and applying for a job there.

I was working part-time creating a pilot project in organisational culture development for the management teams. If they were satisfied with the results the project would be extended. On the last day of my last workshop there was a meeting with all the employees. The oil crisis had hit them hard and they needed to start downsizing. As an external consultant I was the first to go. I was heartbroken. I thought I had finally got back on track just to find myself on the bare ground again.

My husband was safe for a while since he was in a bigger project, but there were forces that wanted that to end as well. We lived every day after that in uncertainty of when we had to leave. I couldn't apply for a job in London or Norway since our stay could be anywhere from 6 months to two years. Living in uncertainty is part of the game and the flip side of being an expatriate.

I continued my journey towards a strong body and mind by taking deep dives into research and books on neuroscience and meditation. The education I had gained from experience was confirmed and gave me a deeper understanding of the processes that creates and preserves energy in the body.

I went to international workshops with Dr. Joe Dispenza and acquired more knowledge on neuroscience and how to change thought patterns, belief systems and behaviour. I felt that I was getting closer to being in sync with my inner voice. The voice I had ignored for so many years in my effort to be a perfect mom, a perfect employee and to please others.

I was participating in a research project run by the HeartMath Institute in one of the several workshops I was attending, when my curiosity kicked in. I wanted to learn more about this method. The similarity with Kouksundo breathing was astonishing to me. I knew breathing patterns had an impact on the neurophysiology of the body and hence the stress level, but with their biofeedback system I could actually see how well I was doing and watch my progress. I was thrilled. What was new to me though was the heart-brain connection. This is the understanding that the heart actually sends more signals to the brain than the brain sends to the heart. This was not something I had learned as a student in my anatomy, physiology or neurology classes. The fact that these heart signals have an effect on emotional processing, attention, perception, memory and problem-solving was big news to me. Yet again, knowledge is fine, but it is the practice that gets the job done.

At that time my motivation was wobbling with so many things to remember and new routines to adjust to. Yes, I had learned about changing thought patterns, but it was easier said than done. Without a job I started to feel miserable and useless again. Even though on some days I fell into dark thoughts, I did not fall into the deep dark abyss I had been in before. I was stronger, now I had the knowledge and experience of climbing up into the light. That experience was much needed when the sad news came.

The message came on a warm and lovely summer day in London. We had to leave and that gave us only 4 months left. At this time I felt I had been away for so long that I wasn't sure I wanted to go back. I was afraid old beliefs and convictions would re-emerge and that I hadn't changed as much as I thought. I knew I would need all my knowledge and experience on my return to my home country.

Homecoming

Moving back to Norway was harder than I had imagined. Thinking Norway was my home turf, I underestimated the culture shock coming back after over 7 years abroad.

All my previous experience and knowledge kicked in and gave me the energy to do what I had been doing for the last 8 years, readjust to new situations and build myself a new life. I started redefining my goals. I had reached my goal to achieve high energy, good health and strength in body and mind. Now it was time to create my dream life.

I knew my competence and expertise, but at the same time I acknowledged that I was a novice in some areas. Where to start? Is this the right place to start? Is this the right thing to start now? So much to learn and so much to experience. This is what it is like living in the unknown and trusting the Universe. This is what it is like being curious and adventurous. This is me. I am back!

I had gone from being completely burned to the ground to rising like a Phoenix from the ashes. I went from being true to myself, to losing my connection, to finding my way back again.

I would never have believed it if anyone had told me 10 years ago that I would start my own business. I would have laughed and said they were out of their minds. But here I am, happy as a clam at high water looking forward to what the Universe will do to surprise me.

Are you in a place where you can't see the forest for the trees? Do you feel blinded by all the problems that are piling up? There is hope. Hope means to have faith. When you choose to have hope for yourself then you choose to have faith in yourself. Faith builds mountains, stone by stone.

Faith in the process led me to the right people and the right places. Trust in the process gave me the internal knowing of what it feels like being in alignment with my true self.

Here are some of the paths that will be helpful on your journey.

B – R – E – A – T – H – E

Breathe

Lay on the floor with your hands below your belly button. Feel your belly move slowly and steadily up and down in a rhythm that feels natural for you. Take a 5 second active inhale and an active 5 second exhale. Do this for 5 minutes and increase gradually so you can manage 15 minutes. When you are ready, try sitting upright and increasing the length.

Relax

Relax, surrender and enjoy the now. It is the now that counts. The past has happened and the future is unknown. The only thing that is certain is the NOW. Start your day by finding feelings of gratitude and create an intention to have a beautiful day.

Emotions

Emotions are the language of the body. Learn the language of the good feeling emotions. What does appreciation feel like? Do you remember? Close your eyes and reactivate that feeling by remembering. It takes some practice in the beginning, but don't give up.

Anchor

Decide what feeling you want to anchor. Chose a suitable anchor; either physiological (body position, touching a body part, etc.) or mental (image, movie, etc.). When you feel the wanted feeling, apply your chosen anchor. Repeat until it works for you.

Thoughts

Be aware of the thoughts that pop into your mind. If it feels farfetched to think positive thoughts then go general. Make statements that you feel you can believe in. Practice this every day and be patient with yourself. It takes time to change thought patterns, but do it one thought at a time.

Healing

Speaking from experience, I can say with confidence that healing emotional scars happens from within. Practice breathing slowly and add regenerative emotions every day. Start with 5 minutes a day and gradually progress as your stamina develops. Have trust in the process.

Envision

Create a vision board or use a treasure box to save pictures of your dream future. Keep it close and look at the pictures as often as you can. Keep them active in your mind and enjoy the feelings they create.

"The secret to life is to fall seven times and get up eight times". ~ Paulo Coelho

About the Author

Berit Bosdal is an experienced facilitator, working to bring resilience and mental robustness amongst students and adults by using mindfulness, NLP and HeartMath techniques.

Being a physical therapist, HeartMath coach and holding a Master's degree in Applied Organisational Psychology, she understands the importance of the body mind connection.

Berit is passionate about the connection between neuroscience, quantum physics and spirituality, and combines different modalities to empower her clients to create and build a stronger mental resilience. Through her work she contributes to help others stretch beyond their perceived selves, discover their true power and transform their lives.

She works with individuals, groups and organizations offering 1:1 sessions, mentoring and facilitating workshops. If you are eager to increase your resilience and set sail towards your expanded future self, Berit will be honored to guide you on your journey!

Please reach out with any questions or comments to: b.bosdal@gmail.com

You can also find Berit on LinkedIn: www.linkedin.com/in/beritbosdal/

The Small Voice Within
by Cynthia J Harrison

She slipped on her satin lined red rose power dress, and fixed her long dark curly mane into coils for an appropriate updo. From wild flow to sophisticated and presentable. This day had significance for her as a senior social worker and therapeutic specialist. She was to go into battle for 3 young girls in foster care, an advocate for the sisters to stay living together.

Yet the overall magnitude of this day far outweighed anything she could ever have imagined.

Early that morning the phone rang, stopping her heart in the moment. Something was wrong, very wrong, her bones felt the chilling urgency. The voice on the phone confirmed the felt sense within her body, saying that her young one was on the way to hospital and may not survive.

As a mother she went into a moment of panic as her mind tried to digest the information. Yet as an ex soldier, her training helped her to gain control and go into action. These roles have been her defenders most of her life, yet rarely for her own child, not since the original battle of her right for life 26 years prior.

This was the second mobilisation rescue mission!

Through the tears that streaked her makeup and soaked her dress, she went to share the happenings with her family then dove straight back into the task at hand; to book a flight, call work, grab some clothes and go to the airport. Everything was dropped to assist this young one.

The waves of emotion ebbed and flowed with this forced shift in consciousness. She was immersed in a world where people were busy completing their daily tasks, all while not knowing if she would ever hold her baby again.

She was composed, yet the tears continued to sneak through her barriers as the cab drove to the airport, trickling down her face again as she checked in to the flight. The wait created knots in her stomach and pain in her chest. She breathed it through and out via the Dragon's Breath, while holding her little fingers to assist her heart energy.

One small relief was that her sister, the young one's aunt, would be at her side soon. This knowledge helped provide some emotional regulation, as the mother role was being covered until she could get there.

On the flight her spiritual practice held ground and showed the way, helping the shock to flow through and out of the body, helping to clear her mind and to discharge nervous system surges. With every text message updating her of the young one's condition, she worked her subtle energies, starting with the channels (meridians) that supported specific organs. She continually held energy for this dear one to find her way.

This was a fight for life reminiscent of earlier battles to live. She heard again that voice of potentiality, the gentle whisper of knowing from a place of divinity which showed there was more to come…

To feel or not to feel?

She can feel her heart now, the actual energy of the compression and expansion. To feel again, to really feel with every cell and point of charge in her body, to sense the pain, suffering, joy and bliss of another within her systems. Life has been a grand journey of discovery, because as a child she was a sensitive and felt it all. What got her through?

What got her through was her body! The body, her vehicle that she abused, poisoned, hurt, neglected, and starved, has seen her through all these years. Many times that body, her precious vehicle, had reached fatigue and then burnout. Her body remembered — our bodies always remember.

Where she fought and strived for recovery of her Self, often the challenges and threats were so overwhelming that as she fought them it all expanded, until she would just inwardly collapse. She spent years walking around without emotion in the survival state. She knew that feeling — or non feeling — very well, where you're in the world but not of it. Going through the motions, but with a dulled spirit and a numb heart.

Her body's score

At age 12 she was already unconsciously trying to exit!

Her behaviours were a plea for help, which escalated to the point of having to be taken to emergency on more than one occasion. Where did this desire to be free come from?

And free from what? Free from confinement, indifference, the guilt or shame so subtly yet regularly piled on from society?

Well, her little body would feel the pains and emotions of many in the world. How could she settle this, how could she just 'be'? Numbing the body wasn't so hard, this tends to occur as the nervous system can no longer work to recover as it once had. Yet there was a psychic pain, a suffering so deep within that she wondered if it was even hers.

by age 12 she was self medicating with whatever she could get her hands on; pills, alcohol, cannabis. Escaping 'All' for small moments of time, and gaining freedom from any imagined or real constraints. The behaviour whispered for help, sending signals that something was not right. Over the next few years this escalated to the soul screams that only she could hear. It was through her actions that she told her story.

She wanted to live but didn't know how. Risking life and limb in daredevil acts of rebellious poisoning and chemical concoctions onto her not yet mature physiology, luckily rescued by concerned bystanders. But what baffles her to this day is why no one ever spoke, no one ever asked her 'why' she did those things nor how she felt.

She would survive one ordeal then move on, showing her time and again that she was not important, she was not valued, and she was definitely not seen nor heard.

Those around her were in their own tornado, being hit with shrapnel and debris from their own lives. Yet she was blessed, she had been blessed! Touched by the hand of the

Beloved, or as the nuns told her, a star had shone down upon her.

Pregnant at 15, to a young man who is loved to this day. Yet the world would not stand for this, she knew from a deep internal knowing that it was not safe to tell anyone. Sharing only with one friend, they would get information from the health centers by catching the bus to town and collect pamphlets. There was no Google back then. Gathering information, they read and studied, making sure she was on the right track with vitamins and a good diet.

Literally, weeks prior the girls would go into town for very different reasons! They would binge eat hamburgers, milkshakes, sweets - and within the hour purge it all. We know it as bulimia now, then it was how they kept their body shame under control. So with the harmful ways they treated their bodies, pregnancy was a life rope!! She had been thrown a way out of the deep dark dungeon of self abuse, out of one fight for life into a very different one.

Accepting what she considered to be a great calling, she chose to keep her young one, the choice had always been to fight for life, this life within. It was through the inner voice guiding her of what was needed that she trusted and kept walking. Wearing oversized clothes and a large winter coat, she concealed the pregnancy for seven and a half months. She changed her behaviour and lived a clean life, truly saying 'yes' to the responsibility. For if she was found out any earlier there would have been a forced termination. Her well meaning mother who was determined to help, sent her to a home for unmarried mothers soon after she found out.

Freedom and rights were taken yet again, however she was determined to rise.

Kept in shame, hidden from the scrutiny of societal bias around age and marital status,

with no communication with the past, and no mobile technologies, she was isolated. As a creative she painted silently in the tiny room to adjust to the circumstances and pass the time. Finishing her education by correspondence under the mentorship of the nuns who ran the facility.

Her physical needs were met, they even booked her in to start the birth process (be induced) at 8am. It was all arranged and the nuns drove her to the hospital. A red rose bud was placed in her hand by one of the nuns who said by the time it opens you will be a mother. She holds that beautiful gesture in heart to this day, and the dried rose in her journal.

Mamma don't preach, I'm keeping my baby

The epidural and birth trauma left her unable to leave the bed, and her baby was immediately taken to be washed and weighed, they said. Exhausted physically and emotionally, she lay immobile wondering what was happening.

She was given something to eat and taken to a new private room, still without her baby. The only visitors were her mother, a Benedictine monk, and a nun with a determined social worker who was trying to gain her parental rights for adoption. She saw she was on her own, no one was standing for her, and no one heard her heart. Still her strength rose in determination, demanding to have her baby to feed, and to know.

'HELP ME' she cried to her big sister, who appeared like an angelic being in the doorway of the hospital room. Her sister had found her and could now echo the voice in a way that together they would be heard. Young one was placed beside her, and she wondered 'what had they done to you'? Looking at her long fingers, and dark hair with a full heart, she was here! Finally, little one was here. With an extended breath she gazed into this new vision, bonding with her little one who was finally in her arms.

Soon after, the nurses moved her into a ward with 5 other mothers and babies. Treating her with contempt, they had to assist her, but it was with few smiles or real care. One nurse took her under her wing though, and because she lacked parenting experience, the nurse organised for her to go to a mother craft home. However it was another archaic facility, the babies were held in the nursery and only out when due for feeds, to be washed or weighed.

Parenting confidence was gained at that home, still there was a feeling that arose of how these clinical settings impacted the children. It was emotionally distressing. No visitors, it was another lonely place. She ate by herself in the big dining room, watching families interact, and would then go back to the nursery alone. The cleaner was a friendly face, a relief in a world where everything was so controlled and sterile.

Many of the mums were not there voluntarily, the court mandated they be there or they would have their children removed. Tense vibes from the watched and monitored, every moment was a fight to stay strong, to get out and begin a new life together.

Once released would the shame reinforced daily fade away, and would they be accepted in society? No! Living in a fish bowl environment of being observed and critiqued, she became a hoop jumper, making sure there were no concerns anyone could report. She was sure the tension and stress of being kept in social isolation with limited opportunities for attachment impacted both her and her little one.

The scrutiny and public judgment became her perfectionism, she felt she had to prove not just good enough, but better than, to be seen as an okay mother. The tensions eventually appeared as anxiety, and later in life this looked like an over achiever with a thirst for knowledge. This alchemised within her to become her treasure, the ability to assist those ostracised in life, and help gain power back. She became the voice for many people, all ages, the most oppressed in our society. She wasn't heard! But she went on to assist other voices to be loud and clear.

26 years later they found themselves in a sterile monitored environment once again, isolated from family and not knowing if all would be well. The alchemy of the past melting away from the charged compression of that life, to change form for a new kind of strength, a resurrection of sorts.

In her body she felt the internal reverberation of a knowing that this young woman has divine work to do. A knowing in her mind's eye and a hearing of the ear of the heart, an energy that moved through her whole being as if it spoke to every cell. It was clear! Young one would be ok, there was a road of recovery ahead, yet she was shown it was to be 'recovery'!

Energy medicine was a large part of the healing each day. Sitting in the park with young one's dog accessing the sacred heart, a process for support with holding the pain and heaviness of the day. This was the time she could break down and through. Not having to stay strong for others, she could cry out her despair and offer it up via the sacred heart. This became her ritual, each day focussing on just one system to work, clearing and strengthening, holding points and protocols for alignment of the subtle energy systems. Working the shock points and any major concern the nursing staff had for the day. Each evening she sat in nature, feeling the days weight and offered it up into transition, transforming it into love, in and through the sacred divine heart. This was her super power, to stay present and in a state of openness and love, no matter the pain.

The resurrection of both mother and daughter from their comfortable nests to rising from the burnt ash like the great phoenix! Now they fly with a vision of what is important and possible, no more living in the shadows of shame, and having freedom dictated, we moved back into our respective worlds, as awakened empowered women.

Pregnancy saved her/my life, having the responsibility to bring this child into the world for her to do her sacred work, of healing and assisting people in their transitioning from birth to death. Fully recovered, a year later that spark was thrown forward just as she/I had been shown in that time of deep distress and uncertainty. Young one became fully vibrant and answered her call to be responsible for the raising of her own three children, with a loving partner and a career as an intensive care nurse.

~~~

Trauma can be a portal for our evolution, a way to be still enough to hear the inner voice guiding, and this small voice spoke to me in times of my deepest soul ache. Showing me my courage and strength, reminding me that we all have resilience to come back from pain, despair or loss of freedoms. Yet at the same time there are days where I have learnt to let go and not be focused on being resilient, or even surviving, and just 'feel' the language of my body Re-Membering; and to deeply listen to what she has to say. From all of these experiences, the ability to be with my full body sensations, to feel them and be present with the Self is the most precious jewel. To know The Self enables a kindness and love of her, a gentleness you would have with your most beloved one. This saves our lives, it is this connection that saves us and is the sacred elixir I bring back from the dark to share.

I AM not being resilient today
No!
I won't be strong and push the pain away
I refuse to numb the hurts inside
Just to feel like I can stay alive.

Yes, I am refusing to be resilient today!

I will swim in the thickness of loss and betray
Feel every moment my body wants to say,
how she has been impacted, and now needs to lay

I won't be here for anyone today
I will be with my body, listening
to all she has to say.

Ask yourself is it more resilience I need, or more
recovery and self compassion?
Freedom is from the inside out...

About the Author

Cynthia J Harrison is the Founding Director of Rhombus Healing Arts in Perth, Australia. She is a Bio Field Science and Eden Energy Medicine Certified Practitioner, with degrees in Anthropology, Social Work, and Visual Arts.

Specialising in human behaviour she focuses on the evolution of the human, physically and energetically – offering a complete mind, body, spirit experience. The keys to Cynthia's work are the physiology overlaid with the energetic understanding of stress and complex trauma for conscious evolution. Knowing the nervous system responses and behaviours that result are core to many illness, disease, and discomfort.

An inventor and visionary artist, she creates interactive opportunities for wellness education and self empowered healing experiences.

To support your nervous system health and wellness go to:

www.rhombushealingarts.com or visit my FaceBook page: Facebook.com/Rhombushealingarts/

Follow me on Instagram @CynthiaJaneHarrison

Twelve Steps of a Recovering/Discovering Adult Child
by Ann Marie Wyrsch

I would like to paint a scenario depicting what it means to be born and grow up "under the influence." You might ask, "Under the influence of what?" All children grow up under the influence of parents or persons who provide them with what they need to survive, or they would not survive. They would die. The influence I am talking about is the influence of unreality, of denial.

Many years ago, a little girl was born into a family with a normal need to experience basic rights as a human being. Her parents did the best they could to provide for her needs, often at great cost to themselves. However, they had not experienced their own basic rights as children. They could not give her what they did not have themselves. Her parents suffered from the diseases of Alcoholism and Codependency. The little girl grew up under the influence of these diseases. She needed to see her parents as perfect because she counted on them for her survival, and so she began to deny reality and mistrust her own experience.

This little girl developed much pain on the inside that she carried into adulthood. She explained the pain by believing that there was something very wrong with her. Denial made it possible for her to not see the truth. She learned early not to see real pictures, about herself or others.

Feelings of fear, sadness, and anger would have overwhelmed her if she had seen real pictures. It was not safe for her to let herself know the truth.

Denial kept her safe, but it limited her greatly. Webster says that denial is "a restriction on one's own activity or desires." So, although denial was helpful to protect her from reality then, denial later caused her to restrict her own activity and desires. She developed the disease of Codependency, which affected every area of her life.

These "Twelve Principles of Codependency" synthesize what growing up "under the influence" translated to in adult life for this little girl.

1. I need to control people and events to provide some predictability and to protect myself from what would feel like overwhelming fear, anger, and sadness. I need to see myself as a victim and focus on others always.

2. I am my own higher power and I need to try harder to achieve and succeed, or get others to achieve and succeed so they can take care of me.

3. I see God as judging and punishing and I better keep on His good side so He will do my will.

4. I create an idealized picture of myself as perfect to get love, and still do not feel good enough. I blame others and myself for whatever goes wrong.

5. I must keep my thoughts and feelings to myself lest others find out how inadequate and confused I feel sometimes, and how terminally unique I am.

6. What has happened to me up to now has no effect on me and I can handle it alone.
7. I have to maintain the status quo because change is terrifying. If I could change others then things would get better.
8. I feel responsible for all that has gone wrong in my family, my school, and the whole world. And I think everybody notices what I do or do not do.
9. I kept trying harder to make it up to others for all the pain I thought I had the power to cause them. At the same time I blamed them for all the pain they caused me.
10. I continued to see what I wanted to see only and not real pictures because then I would never be "wrong" and I would rather be right than happy.
11. I sought to ignore my inner wisdom and look for answers in a relationship, a book, seminar, seeking to avoid personal responsibility whenever possible.
12. Maintaining rigid denial as a result of these steps, I tried to take care of everyone else.

What this little girl now knows is that her family was not perfect. Her parents did the best they could despite the reality that they suffered from the deep and pervasive diseases of Alcoholism and Codependency. They did not know there was a problem, and certainly not what the problem was. She also knows that there was nothing basically wrong with her. She is a normal human being who learned some non-constructive patterns. These patterns are something she learned, and therefore something that she can unlearn and relearn!

Because of the unhealthy patterns, however, she does have the disease of Codependency. The disease of Codependency is now understood as a primary disease from which recovery is possible. I want to share the story of this little girl's recovery because I know it well. It is my story. I am the little girl.

I did not know for much of my life that there are always alternatives, because I saw life from only one perspective. I became a seeker when I first learned that life can be different and richer. As I sought, I learned to trust myself, my source of Life, and the Universe so that now I can use every experience as an opportunity for growth. I now believe recovery from Codependency can be as profound and comprehensive as the wounding is deep and pervasive. The sharing of other recovering adult children helped me start and continue this journey. My personal and professional lives have taken on new meaning and fullness. I want to share with others the hope that was shared with me.

I have some basic assumptions about people, and what I think being a whole human person includes. You may have different assumptions and use your assumptions as a basis for considering what I say. I am aware that even as I articulate my beliefs they continue to evolve. I outline for you here my assumptions:

Each of us has within us the source of life given us by our Creator, and we have a right to be.

Each of us has a right to be fully human, and to feel all our Feelings: including gladness, sadness, anger, and fear.

Each of us has the right to be a separate individual, and to be unconditionally accepted and loved as we are.

Each of us has the right to achieve our unique potential in all areas: spiritually, physically, emotionally, mentally, and socially.

Along with every right there is a responsibility, and a task to achieve that responsibility. My childhood wounding included not accomplishing the tasks to live out my rights. I did not learn to use, or have surrendered, my personal power to connect with the source of life within me and to be responsible for myself. I did not accomplish the developmental tasks of growing up.

I was not aware of what my rights were, nor did I learn the skills to experience them. I made early decisions that limited my freedom to experience these rights. This included the right to be, to feel, to know who I am, and what I want. I learned to negate my own inner wisdom and look to the outside for answers. I have re-decided I want to be loved unconditionally, and to achieve my full potential.

It is not easy, but it is never too late to have another chance. I can still accomplish these tasks. One difference from the first time around is that it is now too late for parents or someone else to provide me with the nurturing I did not get in childhood. My parents tried to give what they had not received and it did not work. This pattern repeats from generation to generation. The cycle is interrupted only when individuals choose to recover and do what it takes to do so.

I can begin the healing. I can learn to give this nurturing parenting to myself. I could not have done it for myself the first time around because I was too little. I can do it now because I have learned how to give nurturing to others. The monumental challenge is to re-decide that I have not only a right but a responsibility to give it to myself.

I can give myself permission to learn what I did not know and use the resources and help that are available. I no longer have to do it alone. I have people who can guide me to use tools and skills to accomplish skipped developmental tasks, and who can provide support for me. I can learn to trust the source of life and growth that is in me. I had learned to deny or negate it. I thought I should know something I had not yet learned.

I learned that the twelve steps of Co-dependence I outlined earlier are a sure fire way to a life of pain and misery. I relearned that Twelve Steps of a Recovering/Discovering Adult Child are a dependable path to a life lived to the full.

Twelve Steps of a Recovering/Discovering Adult Child

1. I admitted I am powerless over people and events outside myself, and I realized my past affected me but I need no longer be a victim.

2. I came to believe that a power greater than me lives within me and within others and can restore personal power.
3. I have decided to turn my life over to the care of God, asking for an ever-truer understanding.
4. I became able to see real pictures about me and to accept myself unconditionally.
5. I experienced the freedom that comes from sharing the truth about myself with God, other persons, and me.
6. I became ready to let God show me how past patterns are affecting me, and I accepted my unhealthy and healthy patterns of thinking and acting without judging myself.
7. I began to let God teach me more healthy patterns and I opened myself to what I am to learn in each of my experiences.
8. I made a list of the persons with whom I have unfinished business.
9. I finish this business in a manner constructive for me and for them.
10. I review each day for unfinished business so I can acknowledge it and complete it at the appropriate time.
11. I seek to increase my conscious contact with God by setting aside specific time to listen, alone and with others, and by always striving to listen to my inner wisdom.
12. I practice these principles as I live life ever more fully, co-creating my life with God to achieve my unique

destiny spiritually, physically, emotionally, mentally, and socially, ever willing to share what I have learned with others.

Regarding: personal power

Before recovering I believed that the church had all the rules. When I became a nun, I was told that if I followed the "rules" I would be guaranteed Heaven. That was just what I wanted, a guarantee. I did not know what personal power was.

What I was looking for was safety and structure so I would not make a mistake. Responsibility terrified me and I wanted God to take care of me. However, I was still not able to be willing to let go of controlling how I wanted God to fix me. I did not trust that God loved me because I did not think people did. I stayed stuck for a long time because of my fear of what would happen if I trusted God to guide me.

In recovery, I have experienced the source of life within me, and still call that source God. I know now that God is not only "out there" but in me and in others.

I used to look in a book for the meaning of Jesus' words: "I have come that you may have life and have it to the full." Although I could always see meaning and purpose in my life, I felt as if life was a pain that I needed to survive rather than an experience to enjoy. I longed to feel loved and to be able to love. I was so wrapped up in myself that I could not do either.

Through growing physically, mentally, emotionally, and socially, I believe I have been able to grow spiritually. As I live the above principles, I see my purpose as that of expanding my capacity to love, and to live life ever more fully as a human person. That brings me back to the rights that I shared earlier. As I accomplished the tasks of healing ever more, I have come to experience those rights. I live life ever more to the full, and feel confident that I will continue to grow in every area to achieve my unique destiny.

A major part of my healing was finding and claiming my own inner child and giving her what I had learned so well to give to others. That child has become very precious to me. I have, with the help of many others, provided her with what she needed to claim her right to be, to feel, to be separate and to give and receive unconditional love. I now accept, with her help, responsibility to co-create my life with God.

I learned I can take care of her and not every other person in my life. by sharing my story and my tools with others, I can help them to find and re-parent their own inner child and experience some of the same rewards. The little girl who needed to see her family as perfect can now see more perfectly, real pictures, as they are. She can appreciate herself and others in a whole new way. She can take risks to grow. She has been born again into awareness and freedom of choice, and no longer had to keep herself buried in denial.[2]

by the time that little girl turned fifty, she had come home to herself. She was able to see options and was open to what the next step would be. Two years later, wanting to share her recovery, she started an Al Anon meeting for Adult Children of Alcoholics. Through a series of serendipitous events, a man came to the second meeting. Turns out that they were meant to share their lives as husband and wife and fell deeply in love. She left the religious order in good standing to follow a new vocation. They married six months later and continued the journey of living and loving more fully. This wounded little girl received the gift of living ever more fully, and was able to share it with another human being.

Using all of her professional education and lived experience, and now with the love and support that she experienced in this relationship, she developed an educational/experiential program for adult children of alcoholic and other dysfunctional families that she named the Recovery/Discovery Series. The program lasted twenty weeks, two hours a week. In a five-year period over three hundred adults recovered from dysfunctional patterns and discovered new skills to live life more fully.

---

[2] This chapter was abstracted and slightly altered from a longer story, with the same title, for adults who grew up in a family with the disease of alcoholism or other dysfunction.   It was written in 1986 and not previously published.

After five years, there was yet another stage of growth to be shared for this couple. Her husband was diagnosed with End Stage Renal Disease. She accompanied him on a five-year journey that included dialysis and a kidney transplant. The transplant failed and dialysis was resumed. He died at home as he wanted to, and the love lives on. She continues to be grateful for all that this journey has unfolded including the depth of joy and sorrow that was, and is, a vital part of living fully.[3]

You may be one of the fortunate people who have already started the journey into recovery. If you are, I invite you to join me in gratitude for experiencing life ever more "to the full." If you are one of the people who is contemplating whether it can ever be different, I invite you warmly to take a risk and go for it. Although your story may be somewhat similar, or very different, recovering and discovering is possible and well-worth whatever effort it may entail to work on it.

---

[3] This section was added in 2019 as a brief epilogue.

About the Author

Ann Marie Wyrsch was an ANA Certified Clinical Nurse Specialist from 1981 until 1997. She retired in 1993 but continues to have a passion for raising awareness of the serious consequences of growing up in a family with alcoholism or other dysfunction, and above all, an awareness that it is possible to recover from codependency and to discover new ways to live.

Ann Marie met the selection criteria for inclusion in **Who's Who in American Nursing**, 1990-1991 Edition for significant accomplishment and leadership and was Included in the **National Distinguished Service Registry in Nursing**, 1988.

The highlight of her career was facilitating a twenty-week *Recovery/Discovery* Series for Adult Children of alcoholic or other dysfunctional families from 1986 to 1991. The series included education and experiential processes addressing the physical, emotional, mental, spiritual and social dimensions of Codependency Recovery. During this time more than 300 adults graduated with new skills for living life more fully.

Ann Marie is a lifelong learner and continues to recover and discover!

She can be reached at amwyrsch@gmail.com

Perfecting Your Persistence

Like many of the resilience traits, persistence is a quality we can cultivate, regardless of who we are and what has happened to us in our life. You may not feel as though you are naturally wired to keep going when times are tough, but every human possesses the innate ability to persist. We are hard-wired to fight for our survival from the moment we are born, which is how we make it through any of life's transitions.

The only aspect of life we can control is ourselves in terms of how we respond to external stimuli. It becomes far easier to perfect your persistence when you become more aware of your habitual responses, thoughts and reactions, because then you can slowly start to improve them.

Persistence is strengthened by strengthening your belief in yourself and in your capacity to achieve what you want when it deeply matters to you. It doesn't matter how long it takes you, or how many times you stumble, when you review your past triumphs, it helps you believe in the possibility of future ones more strongly.

If you find it difficult to look back or remember specifics, you might find it useful to reflect on how you feel when you think about something you really want in your life instead. Identifying the feelings you want in your life can also strengthen your persistence, because it helps you to keep moving forwards towards them whenever resistance arrives.

Use the following journalling prompts to help you identify times when you have overcome obstacles. Trust your immediate responses and try not to overthink the exercise.

This will help you to access your subconscious memory, which is what drives 95% of your behaviors.

Persistence Journalling Prompts

1. Think about a time when you defied your own expectations and achieved more than you expected to. What kept you going? How did you feel during this time? How did you feel afterwards? How does it feel to reflect back on this?

2. Think about a time when you managed to stay calm in the face of stress. Can you picture yourself in that moment? What were you telling yourself to help you stay calm? What did you learn about yourself that day? How has this ability showed up at other times since then?

3. Write down at least one example where you strongly believed in yourself, even though others doubted you. What helped you to stick to your belief in the face of other people's opinions? How did you feel about yourself? What does this tell you about your inner resilience and trust?

It can be useful to store these reflections and revisit these prompts regularly to see how your answers change over time as your resilience and persistence increases.

Notice how you feel after completing the exercise and give yourself permission to feel proud of yourself for taking the time to reflect and cultivate your inner persistence power.

Resilience Trait #4
Tolerance + Compassion

Tolerance and compassion are your secret weapons when it comes to developing and strengthening your resilience. The more tolerant and compassionate you are, the less likely you are to be triggered by circumstances outside your control and the less regret you will have about behaving in a way you later berate yourself for.

These traits offer fast-track tools for becoming a kinder, more understanding and less frustrated human. When you start viewing life through the lens of compassion, you no longer fight with aspects of life you have no control over and you stop creating your own inner world of resentment or anger. Realizing that the majority of people you encounter are dealing with their own problems and concerns helps you to create more genuine connections and develop greater emotional intelligence.

The more you develop qualities such as understanding and empathy, the more you free up your life force energy. This means you can focus on constructively creating your life in every moment, rather than reacting and getting dragged along for a ride by your emotions.

To improve our capacity for tolerance and compassion, we need to start by developing this quality with ourselves. The more we understand, accept and forgive ourselves, the better equipped we are to understand, accept and forgive others.

According to the Laboratory of Neuro Imaging at the University of Southern California, the average person has around 49 thoughts per minute (approximately 70,000 thoughts a day!) and 70% of those thoughts are identical with the day before. If you stop to consider how many of your thoughts you are actually aware of, and how many of those are negative thoughts about yourself, you can imagine how powerful it is when you begin consciously developing more compassion for yourself.

When it comes to tolerance, we are generally far harder on ourselves than we are on others. The words we use to chastise ourselves can be incredibly harsh and we need to learn how to find the balance between letting ourselves off the hook and constantly reinforcing our inner belief that we are not good enough.

Can you imagine yourself as a child or as a baby and send yourself unconditional love and acceptance? Can you see how the mistakes we make in life can easily be tolerated and forgiven when we reconnect to our original innocence and imperfection? How much easier would life feel if you adopted this perspective in future, when you notice that you are judging yourself and others?

Remembering that we all want to be loved and accepted can make it easier to be compassionate with others, as well as ourselves, when we see struggle, striving and anger. Rather than letting our Ego react and rise up to defend ourselves, instead we can adopt practices that help us to be more present, notice when we are triggered and then pause before we respond.

Clinical studies show that regular practice of the popular Loving Kindness (Metta) Meditation can do wonders for mood problems and irritability.

You can find a free meditation and take part in the 21-day Compassion Meditation Challenge here: AttunementMeditation.com/Compassion

You can also listen to guided meditations to experience gentle self-forgiveness and self-compassion here: https://podcasts.apple.com/us/podcast/guided-meditations-by-dr-andrea-pennington/id1122001201

Our first story illustrating the huge power of compassion is from an inspiring teacher and health professional, who learned the hard way how to honor herself before giving all her energy away to others. Even when Helga "Gegga" Birgisdottir had created an instrument of happiness she could share with others, she still pushed through until she was forced to press pause. Like so many caregivers and health professionals, her burnout could have been predicted by seeing warning signs such as a lack of fulfillment from a once enjoyable job. What she shares is a moving portrayal of how her journey to meeting her inner self with greater compassion completely changed her life and gave her freedom.

Our second story is from a man who took a long circuitous route to discovering the unique gifts he is here to share. Along the way, Willow McIntosh learned a lot about how *not* to honor yourself and how this negatively impacts your life experience. Having reached a dramatic turning point in his life, he discovered that his greatest route to inner happiness came from reconnecting to his innermost self. The work he does now is testimony to the resilience of that aspect of himself and to how much unfolded for him when he developed greater self-compassion.

The last story in this chapter is my own. I previously shared this in a book called *Life After Trauma*. My story explores how compassion and meditation helped me recover from a draining few months as a full time caregiver to my mother. Now, I have new insights on how illness can set us on a path to new life. I am more convinced than ever that the practice of self-compassion and meditation can help us develop resilience and provide relief for a whole host of other big and small crises.

The Silent Lion
by Helga Birgisdóttir

There I was, crying and sobbing in the Emergency Admissions ward, not as a patient, but as the on-duty Nurse. It was a cold day in the fall of 2017. The time was 2 p.m. and I was alone in the small pharmacy of the ward where I had been working for the past six years of my thirty-five year career at the hospital. While I was picking out pills and putting them into vials I tried to gain control of my feelings, mostly by looking out the window at the grey parking lot, watching the rain and the trees that swayed in the wind. It didn't help much. I simply was not a tree that moved gently and in harmony with life. I broke down. Fury and lack of power consumed me, I was burning inside and my body was shaking. God how I hated this place and my job, a job I had loved in the beginning.

The crying increased, which surprised me as I am not the type to cry a lot. I wanted to melt into the wax on the linoleum floor, to disappear. But because of the large windows I was visible to all. The mask had fallen.

I was scared, alone in an environment that did not understand me! Fog and confusion clouded my brain. I had just returned from the ICU of Psychiatric Ward on the floor below where my daughter had been admitted unexpectedly. My colleagues had refused my request to visit her, following ridiculously stringent rules they refused to bend. I, the main supporter of my daughter 24/7, didn't get any information. I

144

experienced my workplace as an inhumane and colossal rulebook where human values were not at all important. How can a psychiatric system conduct itself like a cruel dictator? How can my colleagues not show compassion? I didn't trust this system to take care of my daughter.

My guilt was blooming. If I had only been around more when she was little, the situation might be different. I felt like a lion in a cage that wants to roar but is afraid to do so for fear of punishment, a lion in a strange and difficult world that has lost all hope for freedom. The silent roar stretched every nerve of my body. I kept crying and was sent home.

Deep inside of me I heard a low whisper of my soul, "Trust and let go". Was this precisely what needed to happen?

Let me save you

The precursor to my crash was cunning. I had unsuspectingly lost control of my own life. I was drowning in the role of the savior that carried responsibility for the whole world on sore shoulders. I was a fixer, and as such, I got a 'kick' from rescuing people — whether they needed it or not. But when I was unsuccessful in my rescue missions I turned into a victim. I was stuck in a triangle of codependency — a savior, a victim, an aggressor — often all three at the same time. My nerves were shaky and the body was not amused.

One day my colleagues measured my blood pressure at 190/120. Wow! The head nurse wanted to take me in a wheelchair over to the Cardiac Ward. Oh, no! Not me. I preferred to walk even though I might drop dead on the way. In the Cardiac Ward the situation improved after a few hours of rest and some medicine. Two days later I reported back to work, in good shape, I thought. Pain in the musculoskeletal system, irregular heartbeat, unexplainable fatigue, foggy mind, forgetfulness, heaps of crying, irritation, anger, hopelessness, had all been simmering for years and I the chef, continued to stir until everything boiled over. My solution, to work some more in order to feel better, had failed badly.

Sixteen-hour shifts with little sleep in between had become the norm. I, the workaholic, couldn't say no when called upon. I did try though, promising myself to say a firm 'no', if the phone would ring unexpectedly on a Sunday morning and I had gone to bed late the night before. Did I stand up to it? No. In the few instances I did say no, I strolled around the floor like an alcoholic who needs her next drink. Then I called them back and said I would show up. At the same time I was thinking "only this time", something that would repeat itself time and again.

I felt odd pride over my work ethic and importance. At the same time I wondered what was really wrong with me. I had a Bachelor's degree from the College of Arts, I loved to paint and had a nice studio waiting for me. I was also an innovator and lecturer. My greatest passion was SMILER, the Instrument of Joy. I created it to remind me and others that we are Powerful Creators in our own lives and that the most important thing to do is to listen to one's heart and follow one's dreams, exactly what I myself was not doing.

It had not always been like this. In the beginning I enjoyed my work. The ward I worked on was the Emergency Admissions ward and we received new patients every day, often in a suicidal state. I understood them all to well, being codependent and having experienced emotional suffering personally. Something that came from living in an alcoholic environment most of my life. I was good at my job, however, and it was easy for me to liven people up and spark hope in them. I used unusual methods such as starting discussions on faith, God (the word I use for the loving creativity of life), and the meaning of life, a hot topic that only the hospital priest was supposed to discuss. Most patients longed for such discussions and my grayish humor worked on them like a well designed joy pill. My motto was not to end a conversation until I had seen a smile. I admit I felt good when people thanked me for saving their lives. I mattered.

From good to bad, a gradual decline

Art was my favorite way to bond, and for the first few years there was an art room in the ward where I had my best treatment interviews. Oh my God how I enjoyed those days! The art room was then shut down because of budgetary reasons. Recession and a lack of interest in any treatment options other than medicine became the norm. I had given weekly talks for the patients, but cutbacks shut them down as well.

I also used the NADA acupuncture protocol with good results with people with drug withdrawal symptoms and anxiety. As a certified NLP Practitioner Coach I also guided people towards meditation with good results, but that is hard to do when called upon from many directions. Every minute was used and lunchtime and coffee breaks were restricted. Pressure and passion to save as many as possible resulted in me, not even having time to go to the bathroom.

The job lost the joy it had given me. I had betrayed my values and disregarded my heart. No wonder it flew into screaming disorder when going to bed in the evening, pounding like crazy, then stopping, then beating again. I always had the telephone ready on the bedside table in case I needed an ambulance. I remembered my grandmother's good advice, which I always followed: "Always wear clean underwear in case you end up in a hospital."

I sometimes felt like a traitor and even felt abused as a nurse, when I gave patients habit-forming drugs which I believed did more harm than good. My style was to strike up a conversation and provide a kind, compassionate presence instead of an extra dose of drugs. I was starting to give up and I felt I was fighting a losing battle, against ghosts from a distant past.

It was not well regarded to have opinions that were not in line with hospital policy and the staff almost never spoke about the important feelings, the disappointments and the sorrow from traumatic experiences. Dr. Rachel Naomi

Remen warns of the dangers of this when she says: "People who care for others are vulnerable to burn out – psychopaths don't burn out! We burn out because we allowed our heart to become so filled with loss that we have no space left for care."

As part of the process to become a fully certified NLP practitioner and coach I worked with a coach who regularly advised me to take a vacation. I realized that even though I knew she was correct I simply couldn't take time off. What would people think of me, the great savior? The fear of losing this (distorted) image of my self became stronger than anything else. Nobody would trust me. Everybody would think I was fake!

But God did not abandon me, and following the scenario in the pharmacy it was decided that I would take a vacation and get some rest. Now finally everything went haywire because the shame and my inferiority complex drove me crazy. Me on vacation! Over my dead body! I bent over in shame.

Please God, take my painful shame away

Oh my God – it huuurts! I was on my back not able to move, following a backward fall off a breakwater and ending on a rocky beach. My right elbow was broken (I didn't know it then), some ribs were fractured and my head hit a rock and hurt a lot. Thank God for my thick sealskin cap. As I laid there on my back looking up into the grey sky I felt deep gratitude. My "prayers" had been answered. How often had I not thought I would need to be injured in order to be able to relax? Sounds crazy but what could be better than that to deal with the shame that said I wasn't doing well enough.

The cold was biting, minus 11 degrees Celsius, and I had my insulated overalls on my heels as I had been taking a pee just before the fall. It was getting dark and I was all by myself, without a phone. I couldn't move because of the pain and tried twice to scream for help, somewhat sure that nobody would hear me (it was however a small first step in the direction of asking for help.) My friends were in a summerhouse more than a kilometer away. I managed to stand up holding under my right arm with the left one which I also used to hold my overalls close to my side as I could not get fully dressed. I had to be careful not to falter on the slippery rocks. I remember my mantra which I repeated on my way back to the house: "I am not my body – I am a spirit."

Following old habits I denied my physical situation and didn't go to the hospital until two days later. I needed an operation as my elbow was badly broken. It was pieced together with wires and my whole arm encased in plaster cast.

I couldn't do much, I couldn't drive or wash my hair so I had to ask for assistance for various daily tasks. Too bad I wasn't left-handed. But God always finds a way to teach.

Who would have believed that I would ask my ex-husband to wash my hair! This he did with a big smile.

Yes meant 'no' to me. The day after my surgery I got an email from "The Light" (an organization of people with cancer) asking me to replace someone with a lecture two days later. My own talk was originally scheduled a month later. "Yes, of course."

I remembered I couldn't drive, but no problem, I would be picked up. When the driver arrived, I opened the door — topless. "Please, can you help me get dressed?" It would have been more fun if it had been a man, but hey, you can't get everything.

My lecture was supposed to be about stress. I'm not kidding.

The elbow healed but I wasn't in much better shape than before the accident. The hospital's staff doctor insisted that I attend recovery sessions at Virk, a recovery centre run jointly by the union and the state. I felt like a loser, this was the bottom. Me who had been planning to offer Virk my workshops for their clients. Shame and fear were overwhelming, but big thanks to my soul that could reach an agreement with my ego to try new ways, and to stop this nonsensical hubris.

My little one is my savior

I, who originally had the intention to heal myself, all by myself, found out that this was not possible. I now gratefully received all kinds of support that did me good. I asked my body what it needed to heal and I made some changes in my way of life. Now I go swimming in the cold ocean, have a reasonably healthy diet, meditate, keep up my physical fitness, etc.

The *anger* was the worst. How could I see myself as a good person with all this anger towards the healthcare system? Part of me hated my anger and the accompanying feeling of being a victim. I realized that if I wanted to lower my stress hormones I would need to show this angry part of me some understanding and compassion, as anger is a part of the grieving process and it needs its space. I established the goal to love 'all of me' knowing there were wounds that craved love and acceptance.

Finally, I met my greatest master, myself as a child. Little Helga, nicknamed Gegga, showed a lot of courage when she appeared in unusual circumstances about one year after the accident. Having retreated into a small room to be by myself at a San Pedro medical plant session, little Helga appeared, roaring like thunder and expressing her truth with fierce feelings of anger, fear, loneliness and love. Nothing could stop her voice or the crying that shook my body. I tried to step in with reason and logic, but the little one took the stage. One could feel the power in the childlike innocence and her demands to give and receive love. It was like a sword that cut through my heart and let in the light of truth.

This little master showed me I have the inalienable right to unconditional love and I felt an indescribable feeling of freedom. Freedom to love ME — all of me, freedom to be WHO I AM — all the time.

Two days later as I sat meditating with a picture of myself as a little girl, I asked her what I could do for her. The answer was clear: "I want you to never talk badly about me, I want you to love me, I want you to take care of me."

"You are seen – you are heard- you are loved for who you are." A song with Karen Drucker comes off my CD player just now as I am writing these words. Yes, God is always talking to us, we just have to listen.

I am a gift, so are you

My story is exceptional, but then it isn't. People have different stories of their path to finding self love and you would probably not be reading mine unless you had one of your own. We are always a gift to the world – even though we sometimes feel like garbage. Our lives are never wasted – not for a single moment! We are holy beings and we deserve the best.

God will not let you run forever from your True Self. He might give you a soft kick in your ass now and then, and if you don't listen, even break your arm (if that's what you ask for.) I know now that being confused is part of being human.

I'm deeply grateful for my journey and if I had the choice to dismiss any of my past experiences I would say, "no thanks. " I have emphasized to people to listen to their heart and to follow their dreams, even if I haven't always done so. *"Betrayal of yourself in order not to betray another is betrayal nonetheless. It is the Highest Betrayal"* as author Neale Donald Walsch says. I said *"My soul is not for sale,"* and WOW! The feeling of freedom was stunning.

I still have the same passion as before my crash, a passion to support others in experiencing happiness and love. The difference now is that I trust others can care for themselves and thus I do not need to "save" anyone. It gives me immense joy to share in a creative way my knowledge and experience. I do that with SMILER, by lecturing, teaching, and with private therapy. I also use my art, which nourishes both me and those who appreciate it. I have humane demands on myself and I don't need to feel completely whole to shine. Have you ever heard the moon say "Sorry, I can't do any good now, I'm just half full"? Accepting myself in every moment is freedom and that's how I connect to the love and joy in my essence.

FREEDOM is God's greatest gift. To be able to create, to keep trying, to find out what works and what doesn't in order to realize true happiness. Thank God life goes on, and when there are 'downs' the 'ups' will soon follow.

As SMILER says; "You're a Powerful Creator with your thoughts, words and actions!"

Be gentle with yourself.

About the Author

Helga Birgisdóttir (Gegga) is the CEO and Creator of SMILER the Instrument of Joy. Gegga's overall message is that *You are a Powerful Creator*. Her book, *Smiler Can Change it All,* includes inspiring messages of how each of us can access our inner power to create more joy, love and happiness in life.

Gegga has a broad spectrum of education and experience within health care, personal development and art. She has worked at the National University Hospital of Iceland, both as a nurse and a midwife for 35 years. Gegga is a certified Neuro Linguistic Programming (NLP) practitioner and coach and she is trained in the NADA acupuncture protocol for drug and alcohol detox. She is also a facilitator of *The Work* of Byron Katie.

Gegga has a Bachelor of Arts degree from The Iceland University of the Arts. Gegga is a popular lecturer who offers a variety of workshops and private sessions to coach people to get in touch with their inner love, joy and creativity. She combines spirituality, faith and science in a way people find easy to understand. Within the art world she has been active in private and collective exhibitions both in Iceland and internationally.

Gegga is also a contributing author in *Time to Rise*, published by Dr. Andrea Pennington

Connect with Gegga online: gegga@smiler.is

- *www.smiler.is* - *www.gegga.is*

Ownership and the Path to Resilience
by Willow McIntosh

My journey into understanding what resilience, personal success and happiness truly mean to me could not have happened in a more round about fashion. For me to surrender to who I actually am meant admitting how addicted and obsessed I was to remain stuck, stubborn and essentially unhappy. My journey into my own peace and happiness ironically meant that resilience would come from being relaxed and open to my true nature.

At the start of my journey I figured the more I pushed, the more I suffered and the more I tried, the more resilient I was being. Yet I couldn't have been farther from the truth. My story is one of denial and one that began in the agony of sheer self rejection.

Self-rejection

As a child, I enjoyed a connection to nature that was uncanny. I lived in a flowing, illuminated reality where I could *feel* colors. My enthusiasm for life was expressed in a vibrant way that didn't sit well with the adults around me. So I felt the need to hide much of what I experienced so naturally and powerfully.

I had created a false version of myself, initially for self-protection. But I took that false self with me and hung on to it until it caused me to lose everything. I had chosen to pursue a reality that simply didn't belong to me. In fact I had been trying to fill a cup that wasn't even based in reality. But I had to work it all out for myself.

I knew it was down to me to uncover why I felt so unhappy for so long. The aching feeling in my soul that I just wasn't being the person I knew I was inside. Not living the life and purpose I could sense I am here to share.

I always had a sense of my value. I never lost the baseline of this magical, enchanted beauty within so steeped in love it would regularly cause me to cry deeply at the feeling of its loss. The truth was that nothing was ever lost, it was simply repressed because that reality, that version of myself, wasn't supportive to the false version I was so obsessed with making successful. Or trying to become successful through it.

People say the route to redemption is through finding the answers within. The people who mean it are those who have done exactly that. In my experience there is no other route to true self actualisation and it is a journey I feel we must all take. One that is the unique design of our own hearts conditioning and vibration. It is the journey of all journeys, our own personal Hero's Journey if you will.

We can also choose to refuse this journey for the entirety of our lives. The refusal of which causes that intense pain from our soul that we choose to repress with unhealthy relationships to food, drugs, sex, alcohol and all sorts of behaviour we humans are so good at. It was in this place of deep pain and soul soreness that my story begins.

The beginning of the end

It was a couple of weeks before Christmas, 2009. At 34 years old, I found myself sitting in a waiting room at Brighton Courts, holding my list of creditors that amounted to a six figure debt, having lost my home and my business. I was waiting to see the judge to declare bankruptcy.

Before I take you further into that painful day, let me begin with a little background.

I have always been on a spiritual quest from as early as I can remember and as many of us Lightworkers do, our journeys begin with great trial and adversity. This superpower I had residing in me, the one that was going to be the great redeemer, was pushed so far away from me during my childhood I began my adult life in a state of deep loss. So much so that I did not go to university in the UK with my friends when I turned 19.

Instead, I knew I had to do everything I could to begin my journey to try to recover this thing that I could sense was so important to me. Yet at the time it was like looking into a cave filled with fog. There was such yearning for whatever it was I knew I had to retrieve, but it felt so distant.

For seven years I embarked on a pilgrimage abroad, living on every continent learning, absorbing and challenging myself in every way I could. I lived in meditation centres, went on retreats, stayed with as many learned masters as I could and underwent grueling deep soul work. Driven on and on by this ever growing conviction.

Gradually I began to shed the grieving from the overwhelming losses and events I had endured. As I released vast swathes of grief following yet another 10-day silent retreat or cried until I was utterly spent in the foetal position in the mud, having been 'reborn' from an enduring sweat lodge, I began to feel the fog clearing and a stillness return to me. I began to glimpse with the eyes of an adult what I had embraced as a child. At the time I had no idea it was to develop into the gift I have today and it was going to be much longer before anything made any sense.

When I returned to the UK from my travels I was convinced the only way I was going to get happy was if I became financially successful. So I put these insights I received during my pilgrimage aside and decided on following my Grandfather's footsteps into a career in property development.

They say that life is lived moving forwards but only makes sense backwards. When I look back it seemed as though I had turned my back on the realisations I had uncovered abroad. Yet I realise now that it was all part of a greater plan.

In fact my property development business was the perfect opportunity to prepare me for the work I am really here to do. At the time, though it was all about the promise of success and status. Underneath that, I was trying to buy acceptance from my parents. Underneath that I was really trying to find acceptance and love for myself.

I achieved success financially to some extent over the 5 years since I started the business, and in the time leading up to that fateful day in 2009 I had built a portfolio I jointly owned with my business partner and was due a considerable payout from the business.

Yet there I found myself sitting in that terrible room in the Brighton Courts. Each movement of my Italian shoes echoing back to me from the bare walls as I shifted uneasily. The uncomfortable bench bolted to the floor. My bankruptcy paperwork becoming more and more damp in my cold sweaty hands as I waited for the judge to summon me.

I had chosen to face this alone. I felt so much shame about the loss of the business. Even though it was predominantly due to the economic crisis. I still felt like I had failed.

When I was finally summoned I opened the door into a large office, the musky smell of books and furniture polish. My eyes met with a distinguished man in the later part of his life. A man of presence and position as he called me over to sit opposite his large antique leather topped desk.

I sat down into the same feeling of fear I had felt as a child going in to see the headmaster at school fearing the slipper, or worse, the cane.

In the end the process itself was actually quite painless. I was made aware of the reality of what I was doing, about the coming consequences, and then it was done. As I stepped outside, I felt a sense of relief, a weight was lifting and I acknowledged that a new chapter was emerging.

The next part I am about to tell you sounds a little far fetched, but it actually happened. It's only happened this one time in my life, but it did.

That evening I sat on the step of my cabin looking up at the sky and contemplated what I was going to do next. In my heart I knew what that needed to be. So I looked up and asked the question. No sooner had I finished the sentence a shooting star flew across the night sky.

After leaping about in utter disbelief at what had just happened, it was the calling I needed. The time had come for me to get honest, to get *really* honest about who I was and what I knew I was really here to do. That meant accepting the truth about myself I had uncovered during the time I was abroad.

In the next few weeks I was introduced to a Reiki master who became pivotal in the acknowledgement I needed to make. *That I was born with a difference.* To acknowledge once and for all the acute sensory perception I was living in. The extreme reaction my system had to criticism, to getting tired, to feeling overwhelmed. The unending need I had to fight against what I felt was wrong. Wrong with people, with jobs, with the world, with me. The way my central nervous system just seemed hell bent on controlling me, how it would drive me to constantly look for confirmation everywhere around me that I was broken. When in fact this very heightened sensory experience was to be the very route into the exact opposite of all these things, my truth.

A gift, not a curse

Fifteen percent of the world population are born with a genetic personality trait known as 'Sensory Processing

Sensitivity'. This is recognised as a deeper level of cognitive processing and an increased receptivity to the central nervous system. I can testify to the depression that is caused when this trait is misunderstood and rejected.

A big contributing factor to this is how people are labelled as being too sensitive, and as a part of my work now, my mission is to reframe this into 'High Sensory Intelligence' which is a far more fitting term. This trait in fact affords some incredible advantages, such as heightened levels of empathy, intuition, creativity and visionary abilities.

What began to happen to me was a re-uniting and acknowledgment of this incredible part of me. Through my practise and self engagement, I could feel the sunrise of my own authenticity dawning into my reality. Slowly I began to experience this beautiful connection I had with something greater than me, that I had been so utterly immersed in and so fascinated with as a child. The part of me that was always there, continuously giving me reassuring signs that the answers I was looking for were literally under my nose, residing in my heart.

I came to learn that my real truth, my actual reality was the most stable, powerful, nurturing and joyful reality I could have ever wished for. I simply had to get out of its way and take ownership of the gifts it holds. I had to peel off these layers of habits of continuous self rejection and stubbornness; the version of myself I thought I needed to be to feel safe, loved and accepted.

In fact, the real safety lay in my own self acknowledgment. It became safe for me to be me again. Only through trying this did I break the false belief that I wasn't safe in the first place. It was the pain of my false self trying to defend itself from feeling unsafe that was making me feel unsafe!

So what was happening? What was this awakening?

I was awakening to the innate ability I had to utilise this deeper cognitive processor. I was awakening to the realisation of a connection to a higher reality I was able to access through the heightened receptivity of my central nervous system. This was the dawning awareness into an energetic experience of myself.

I now understood that this experience and my high levels of empathy meant I had a powerful ability to initiate other people with sensory processing sensitivity to experience their own reality into a space of deep self acknowledgment and purpose alignment. I realised that I had in fact been doing this all along with people over the years.

Furthermore, I began to realise the roles I had been playing in business were always about aligning people with a higher vision into purpose. So I began to implement my skills and fascination for teaching, process design and online technology. My ability includes was to activating others into the realisation of their unique high sensory abilities and showing them how they can create highly sought after products and services. In doing so I took my first real client to seven figures in twelve months.

As I embraced this further and further, so my own sense of self began to shift. Suddenly the very central nervous system I had been so averse to gave me access to the most profound sense of connection. The source of my own power, success and happiness was to be accessed through the perception of my heart. This high sensory experience I was living, in secret and in denial, was now the very source of my strength. The gift of intuitive facilitation and Lightworker activation that I had finally embraced gave me access to my grounded, powerful and highly resilient self that was there all along.

So what was the question I asked as I sat on the step to my cabin?

"Shall I pursue a career in facilitating people in the art of finding heart?"

Which in time was to become the name of my first book.

If there is one thing I can leave with you with that I have learned along the way, it is that we are a part of a greater context. Whilst there is great atrocity in the world, we are gradually moving towards good. We only have to look back two hundred years to see the progress we are making.

Each of us has a place and a part to play. If you allow it, nature will conspire to support you. However, you've got to get honest. You've got to allow yourself to be you. No matter what you need to face and overcome to get there.

And it is there that you will find all the resilience you will ever need.

About the Author

Willow McIntosh specialises in facilitating heart-centred healers, coaches and lightworkers to become empowered leaders.

Unique circumstances during Willow's childhood led to the burying of his authentic self and complete misalignment to the work he was destined for. He began to carve his own path of understanding how empathic entrepreneurs with sensory processing sensitivity can learn to use their genetic traits to their advantage. As an adult this led to a lifelong enquiry and practise of learning powerful energetic alignment techniques to re-engage with the authentic self.

Having successfully facilitated the development of seven figure businesses, Willow now specialises in process design and business automation for luminaries and highly empathic business owners. It is the revelation of purpose and authenticity into higher service that he teaches as an author, speaker and facilitator.

To find out more about Willow and his mission to awaken and empower light workers all around the world please visit www.inluminance.com

Recovering from Caregiver Burnout by Andrea Pennington, M.D., C.Ac.

The calm before the storm

I had the pleasure and luxury of creating a deep meditation practice for several years in response to following my heart and moving to France in 2010. Sitting on the beach, meditating in the countryside and becoming grateful for life's beauty became my soul nurturing rituals long before I really needed them. Becoming more mindful and compassionate helped me deal with frequent minor life frustrations — such as dealing with the French administration, traveling to multiple countries with a small child and running a global media company from Europe.

Meditation, QiGong, aerobic exercise and being in nature with lots of sea and sun have helped me stay upbeat and optimistic. I believe they keep the ugly monster of depression at bay, something I experienced for most of my life.

I'll offer my advice to you right up front here — rather than waiting until your life is falling apart, your mental outlook is down the drain or you lose a loved one, I suggest you make meditation a regular part of your healthy lifestyle, so that over time you build up resources to cope with life's many challenges and if you're in need of an emergency rescue, meditation may be just what the doctor ordered.

Mom's Diagnosis: Alzheimer's Dementia

About eight years ago my siblings and I all expressed how obvious it was that Mom was becoming more forgetful and easily confused. Over the last few years each of us saw a dramatic and rapid decline in both her short term memory and daily functioning. It was tough for us to come to terms with the fact that our mother, who had been a sought-after, brilliant physician, was then at the age of 83, asking us the same basic questions every five minutes. To make matters more challenging, Mom is also nearly blind now due to a long history of glaucoma and she is often in physical pain due to arthritis.

In the early stages of her dementia she experienced frequent mood swings. Mom has always been feisty, but soon we watched her go from snappy and irritable to weepy and blue in a matter of minutes. Needless to say, this became quite a challenge for my sister and brother who were Mom's primary caretakers.

A visit to the Cleveland Clinic Center for the Brain led to the inevitable diagnosis of dementia, most likely the Alzheimer's type[4]. Like so many people with a family

---

[4] I say most likely because you cannot officially diagnose Alzheimer's disease without looking at brain tissue under the microscope. Short of a brain biopsy, which nobody living wants to do, the only way to know for sure requires a brain analysis after death.

member diagnosed with dementia, my initial reaction was to jump into rescue mode. As a physician who specialized in longevity medicine, I suggested we bring an arsenal of 'smart drugs' into play. These are the nootropics today's savvy bio hackers take starting in their 20s, whereas my wealthy executive clients began taking in their 40s to maintain sharp focus and to enhance brain function.

We tried a few of the medications approved for dementia which, unfortunately, had a host of side effects that were just unbearable for Mom. One pill got her too amped up. She would stay up all night long talking, and sometimes dancing! Another medication sharpened her thinking but sent her back in time to a period in her life where she owned a medical clinic. She would angrily yell that she was being mistreated and prevented from getting to work where she insisted that patients were waiting to see her. If she was particularly wound up, she could be heard talking to herself, counseling the imaginary patients who she 'saw' in front of her.

My sister and brother alternated caring for Mom for a few years before their own signs of stress and overwhelm became so obvious that I was compelled to step in. It wasn't easy though. Over time my sister had become fiercely protective of Mom and often interpreted any help from me as a sign that she wasn't being trusted to care for her properly. For example, when I offered to fly from my home in the South of France to help them move into a new house, or to take mom on holiday for a few weeks, my sister defiantly said, 'No!' However, things became even stickier when I visited during the Summer of 2015 as it was clear that both my sister and my mother needed a break.

The rescue

I've connected with other caregivers of aging family members or spouses and I now have a greater understanding of how easily our lifestyle and household can crumble around us. Simple things that could easily be fixed are neglected while we care for someone who needs near constant attention. So many of us caregivers put our own needs last on the list — if they get on the list at all!

Though my sister rejected any physical help from me over the last two years I began to doubt my decision to stay away. When I arrived to visit I was beside myself. "I should have insisted," I agonized. I saw the full impact that assuming full responsibility for everything had on my sister. As a single working woman with no husband or other relatives nearby, the care taking role had become too much for my sister. And she rejected the idea of hiring an assistant to help out fearing that they might abuse Mom while my sister was at work. So Mom, who had always been so proud of her beautiful home, was now literally blind to the shabby conditions she lived in. This is when my guilt set in.

My mother was so happy to hug me and her granddaughter when we arrived and she pleaded for us to take her away. I felt so ashamed for not insisting on a visit sooner to unburden my sister from the full-time care taking responsibilities and I couldn't bear to see my mother so confined. So my daughter and I swooped in and agreed to take Mom on a jaunt half way across the map to my home on the French Riviera.

While waiting for Mom's passport to be renewed we spent a month together in the US and treated Mom to several outings and fun excursions. During that month I saw firsthand how fast Mom's memory and physical capacity was deteriorating. She was blind, immobile, confused. I felt sorry for her being now wheelchair-bound due to achy, stiff joints. In my mind it seemed like such a terrible state to be in. I was filled with compassion and felt compelled to do all that I could to both alleviate her suffering as well as provide as many enjoyable, love-filled moments as possible. Plus I wanted my daughter to have positive memories and happy moments with her grandma. So I went into overdrive — dinners, movies, miniature golf and ice cream.

Mom always loved Baskin & Robbins ice cream, in particular the flavor Pralines and Cream. Having left the US nine years ago my daughter had never been to B&R, so while in Los Angeles I decided we'd have a Pennington girls bonding experience. After going through the drama of dressing Mom and putting on her wig and makeup (she was always a proud lady wanting to be seen looking good!) we descended the long flight of stairs to reach the car. I drove with such joy and anticipation as the sun was shining down on Mom's face in the passenger seat.

At the ice cream shop my daughter was filled with wonder at the vast numbers of ice cream flavors — 31 to be exact. As we sat down to enjoy our tasty treats Mom was in

Heaven! I felt so pleased with myself. It felt like a positive accomplishment.

After gobbling down the delicious treats, we piled back into the car to head home, which was only about a 15 minute car ride. I pulled up, parked the car and just as Mom opened the door she says, "You know, I'd really love to have some ice cream."

She had completely forgotten the dreamy, ice-creamy bonding experience we just shared!

Undaunted, I comforted myself and reminded my daughter that even if her mind didn't store the memory, at least her soul could recognize the effort that her daughter and granddaughter made to be fully present and loving.

The descent

Mom was so delighted that she was going to be visiting France again, a country she loved and hadn't seen in over 25 years. Optimistic that the trip to Europe would bring Mom's spirits high, we packed up the wheelchair, her walking stick, medications and boarded our flight. If you think traveling with a small child is difficult, let me tell you, flying with someone who is confused, blind and forgetful is much harder! Needless to say, the plane ride was a horrendous nightmare and only a precursor of things to come. Mom did not believe that she was on an airplane. She insisted that she was in her home as she called out to everyone who passed by her seat. Suspicious that the passengers might be thieves, she tried to climb out of her seat and would reach across the aisle to touch the person sitting there to see who they were.

When we landed in France Mom was so disoriented she refused to leave the plane so the attendants had to carry her off as she resisted and yelled at them. The taxi ride home from the airport was equally embarrassing. She tried to climb into the front seat and begged the driver to let her out. She banged on the windows and called for the police to help her. Little did I know that my attempt to bring her joy and relief was only going to bring her — and me — sadness and misery.

With the time zone difference and Mom being totally disoriented, we stepped into a period of catering to her every need 24/7. Mom's anger and frustration for being out of her comfort zone led her to descend into a child-like tantrum on a daily basis. It's not hard to imagine the consequences: sleep deprivation, physical and emotional exhaustion, depression and yes, resentment.

Drawing on compassion and tolerance, my daughter and I persevered to keep Mom comfortable and entertained. But to no avail. I was worn down by her angry outbursts and nightly conversations with medical patients who didn't exist. Ultimately the fatigue and jabs at my wellbeing were too great. In my mind, I had given everything. My time, home, sleep, money, attention and care had been used and abused, not appreciated nor cherished, by the woman who gave me life. I was hurt by her lack of appreciation for what we sacrificed in having her in our home. Which made me feel ashamed for being so selfish! I was deflated and dejected.

Yet, what did I expect? Wasn't I the one who stepped in, posing as the heroic (codependent) savior, sacrificing everything for her? Was it realistic to think all would be rosy and well? After all, she is the one with a brain that is seemingly disintegrating before our very eyes. She is the one facing the last years of her life totally dependent on others, in pain and confused. Where did the unrealistic expectation that she would or could recognize how much we cared come from? And how could I be so damned selfish?

My refuge — Meditating on compassion

Realizing how bratty my internal dialogue had become, while hiding in the bathroom in shame and guilt, I broke down crying. My refuge and return to sanity came through my practice of meditation, specifically the Mettā, or loving-kindness meditation. Mettā is a Pāli word that involves the desire that all living beings be well. It is more than just a feeling, it is an attitude of friendliness. From a Buddhist psychology perspective, if loving-kindness is directed towards our own suffering then self-compassion can arise, while if it is directed towards the suffering of others then compassion for them can develop.

To practice this meditation we begin by taking a few deep breaths to get centered and quiet. Then we begin with directing loving kindness toward ourselves. Sitting quietly, we mentally repeat, slowly and steadily, the following or similar phrases:

"May I be happy.

May I be well.

May I be safe.

May I be peaceful and at ease."

After directing loving-kindness toward ourselves, the practice involves holding the same kind intention toward people close to us, our loved ones and family. Next we extend the circle of compassionate wishes to people who are neutral, such as the grocery clerk, delivery guy or a random person we stand next to at the post office. Finally, we sit and direct compassion and the wish to ease suffering to difficult people, the ones in our life or in the world who seem particularly difficult to love.

I can tell you from personal experience this practice is profound. Beside the inner transformation that comes from finally being kind toward myself, I have recognized a clear shift in all of the relationships in my life. The loving-kindness meditation has grown in popularity among psychologists and therapists. Clinical research is finding the same results in a variety of different settings[5]. In clinical

---

[5] The benefits of reciting or thinking the simple phrases of the loving-kindness meditation improve love and social connections, too. A study in 2010 showed that participating in a 7-week loving-kindness meditation course helped to expand love and improved health on a personal level for participants.

Cohn, Michael A., and Barbara L. Fredrickson. "In Search of Durable Positive Psychology Interventions: Predictors and Consequences of Long-Term Positive Behavior Change." The journal of positive psychology 5.5 (2010): 355–366

studies this meditation practice leads to an increase in positive emotions over time, which leads to an increase in resilience resources, including mindfulness, self-acceptance, received social support, and positive relations with others.

Becoming more tolerant and compassionate to myself, allowed my heart and mind to reopen to offering true compassionate care to my mother. Through meditation we remember simple advice: just be present; that's the gift. As I eased my grip on internal expectations and released the tension of resisting what was happening, I found greater peace, and so did Mom. Her mood lightened significantly. I stopped telling her that her imaginary patients weren't there. I allowed her to enjoy the idea of being a helpful, caring physician, a role that had given her life tremendous significance. And the tension in the household was magically lifted.

As I relaxed into a solemn acceptance of Mom's condition, I could watch with wonder how she selectively relived certain memories from her early adult life in England. She recounted stories of her time in nursing school in London, the countries she visited, the men she dated (despite her family's disapproval), and the adventure she embarked on with her immigration to the United States. She expressed great pride and satisfaction while recounting stories of her time at medical school when I was just a baby. She beamed with joy and satisfaction at a life lived with no regrets.

Mom often told me how happy she was with her life. Yes, she said she wished there was a man to romance her —

even at age 83! And yes, she wished she had more to give to her children and granddaughter as an inheritance. But she told us, on more than one occasion, that she felt a deep sense of satisfaction and pride that during her illustrious lifetime, she had done "her Master's work" to the best of her ability. She often said, "when I cock up my toes and go to the great Beyond, I shall hear 'Job well done!' And that's all that matters to me now."

The resilient rebound

Through meditation and becoming fully present and accepting of the current circumstances, I came to terms with my own attachment to a desire for her to be 'well' again. I had to let go of my clinging to the vision of the Mom I grew up with and looked up to. A newfound acceptance and appreciation of the frailty of life emerged.

I renewed my personal boundaries and recommitted myself to my own compassionate self-care routines including lots of meditation breaks, hot baths, movies on the couch with my daughter and long walks in nature. Rather than sleeping with one eye open and jumping up every time Mom started chatting, I decided to give in to peaceful sleep and allow her to talk to imaginary people through the night. Instead of rushing home to supervise her every meal and movement, I hired a caretaker to come in during the day so that I could continue my outdoor exercise routine.

Allowing myself time in nature to breathe and reconnect with Life, I slowly let go of the need to 'fix' Mom. And I allowed myself to become mindfully aware and grateful for life.

The resolution

The resolution arrived only a few months later as I returned Mom to my sister's open arms back in America. I was relieved and sad at the same time. I feared that this might be the last time Mom recognized me. She seemed happy to be reunited with my sister, though she didn't realize that she hadn't been away from her for long.

On my last day I pulled out my laptop and we listened to my first TEDx presentation, the one I gave in Monaco about becoming who you really are. She listened with great attention and wonder. After hearing my 18-minute talk she told me that she could tell that I was 'doing my Master's work.' She expressed a sense of pride that was so gratifying to me, especially after so many years of yearning for acceptance and approval.

As I left for the airport the following day and hugged Mom and my sister goodbye I was at peace. I had fully accepted that I had done my best, in the eyes of myself and my soul, as well as in the eyes of Mom and my daughter.

I, of course, clearly saw the many errors of my ways. But I did not have any regrets. The choices I made felt right at the time. Given my own level of awareness and understanding I gave my all, with the best of intentions.

The experience allowed me to connect with my sister on a deeper level as well. And now she knows that she can call on me, even just to vent her feelings. And we both recognize the value in taking time for ourselves and how to laugh or shrug off the sometimes nutty things that happen with Mom. And we know that no matter what, we know that we can get through turbulent times and family crises with true grace and ease.

The update

It has been 4 years since that tumultuous and traumatic summer. When my daughter and I last returned to visit my mother and sister we were fully equipped with compassion, patience and a willingness to be present with Mom as she is **now**. Not carrying expectations or regrets allowed us to visit with her in a joyful and peaceful way.

Armed with lots of her favorite music we danced, we talked, introduced mom to vegan ice cream and we let her share what was on her mind. I was particularly struck by her new acceptance of her condition. She is in an advanced stage of dementia now and thankfully, she is more peaceful, grateful and focused on happy things. It was strange to see her turn down multiple offers to leave the house, have her pillow fluffed or her drinks re-heated. She told us that she was quite comfortable and so very appreciative of our presence.

I was deeply touched that after just a short while she pulled me close to say that she was doing so well that she wanted me to go. I was kind of shocked to hear her say, "You are young, you have your life to live now. You should be out there!" She gestured toward the door. She continued, "I'm doing well, I'm happy you came to visit, but I've lived my life, now it's time for you to go out and live yours."

Once again I felt her giving me permission to live fully and continue my life in France and it brought tears to my eyes. by being present with her without expectation, she returned to the caring mother who wants the best for me.

Even in her fragile state my daughter and I received such precious love and attention, which is what we had intended to give to her. These are moments that have left such a strong impression on me.

The lessons

To summarize but a few of the lessons the summer with Mom taught me.

- Life is precious. This human life is truly a gift to be cherished. We will be wise to live each day authentically, with purpose and always with the intention to give this life deep meaning.
- Life, as we know it, will end. So do not take youth for granted! Everything in this life is temporary and subject to change. We cannot escape pain, sickness, loss or death, so while you're here, nurture your body and brain. Enliven your heart and soul with adventure, love and fun. Savor the pleasurable

experiences without clinging, knowing that all good things must come to an end. And resist the temptation to push away or fix every 'bad' thing. They, too, shall pass.

- Our behaviors determine the quality of our lives. The actions we take and choices we make are what bring forth the fruit of our lives, so be sure to generously choose love and compassion. Practice kindness and forgiveness to yourself as well as others. Cherish your ability to love freely, and often. Mom remembered her greatest loves, travels and triumphs — not the failures. She was able to say she lived with no regrets. Could you do the same?

- None of your possessions, jobs or accomplishments provide lasting comfort or fulfillment in themselves. And at the end of your life, none of them will go with you. So develop an open curious mind and heart while walking without attachment or resistance. Your determined focus on awakened living, serving others and evolving your mind and soul is paramount.

Tools for Building Tolerance and Compassion

The more understanding you have of your own reasons for doing what you do, the more understanding you will have of others. We are all motivated by similar desires and most humans are genuinely doing their best. The more we understand that and learn to celebrate our individual qualities and value, the greater our tolerance levels.

Developing more compassion will benefit your mental wellbeing, as well as make your life run more smoothly. In addition to the Compassion meditation I refer to in my story, which can be found at www.AttunementMeditation.com/Compassion, you can also use the following tools to help you strengthen your tolerance and compassion. Over time you'll find that you are less triggered by others and more in control of your physiological responses.

Tune into the power of your breath

Take the time to breathe, and say a safe, calming interrupt word — like "peace" or "calm." This can help you reconnect to the compassionate side of you that recognizes we are all connected, and we can all use a break sometimes!

To strengthen this, when you say the calming word, press the tip of the thumb of your dominant hand into the centre of the palm of your other hand. This is a calming acupuncture point that helps you to calm your system and also anchor your intention for more compassion towards others.

Rise above your resentments

When you store resentment in your mind, you are giving energy to situations or people that you cannot control or change. This uses up your energy and hurts you far more than it hurts anyone else. Use the following prompts to start letting these feelings go, so that you take your power back by being more forgiving and tolerant of others and yourself.

✓ Are you willing to offer a mental pardon to someone who did you wrong or made you mad?

✓ Can you look at the bullies in your life through the eyes of compassion, recognizing that it is their pain, anger or confusion that causes them to behave badly?

If you find this difficult, can you write them a letter of understanding that acknowledges how much inner pain they must be carrying? You don't ever have to show this to anyone else and you can burn it once you've written it, but this can be an incredibly powerful exercise.

We carry so many self-judgements in our heads and we forget that this is harmful and limits our growth.

✓ Can you give yourself permission to forgive yourself, too?

✓ How would your younger self feel if he or she was forgiven?

Write at least one example of a time when compassion for yourself or another was relevant or appropriate. What can you learn from reflecting on this?

Resilience Trait #5
Optimism

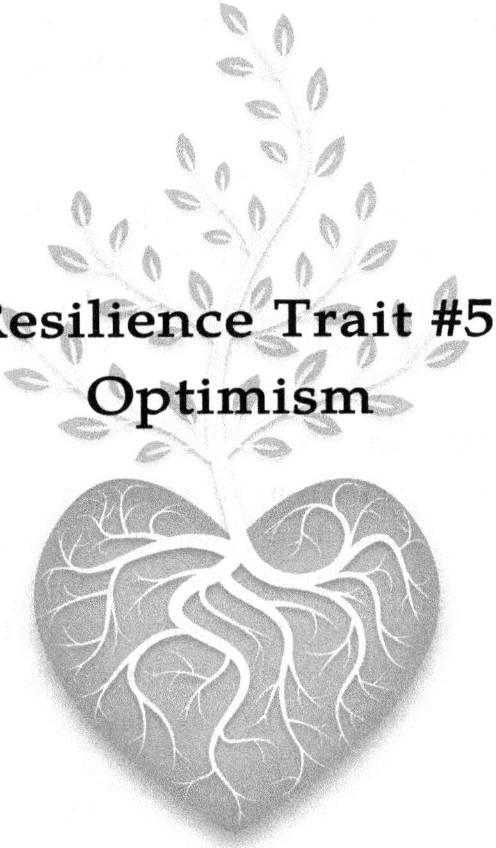

Did you ever see the film Pollyanna when you were younger? If so, you already have a clear image of the ultimate optimist — at the beginning of the film anyway!

Pollyanna's approach to life was to find the good in everything that came her way. She was depicted as an eternal optimist, who lived in a town full of embittered people and eventually her approach to life rubbed off on everyone around her.

It is hard to imagine a resilient person without also seeing them as an optimist, because generally speaking, those who have the ability to bounce back from adversity tend to view life positively. Rather than let circumstances dictate their outlook, optimists believe that they can control their own experiences, and this becomes the lens through which they view their world.

The word Pollyanna is used in modern culture in a more disparaging way, describing someone who is blindly optimistic and delusional. The truth is however, that an optimist has learned the art of reframing, whether knowingly or not. It is merely a matter of perspective, choosing to see situations in a way that boosts you, rather than depletes you.

When we are overcome with doubt, it's easy to imagine that the whole world is against us. To rise above pessimism we can learn to adopt a more hopeful perspective. The good news is that reframing can be mastered by anyone and it is one of the best gifts you can ever give yourself, because it elevates your experience of every day life.

Martin Seligman is a world-renowned psychologist and leading researcher into the field of positive psychology and optimism. His work has contributed to the understanding that we can all learn to become more optimistic, even if we are brought up in an environment that taught us to view life as a long battle you can never win.

Being optimistic is not about wearing rose-tinted spectacles or glossing over difficult feelings. It is a learned skill that means you not only extract more joy from your day, you are more likely to have more days to extract joy from. Researchers have studied pessimists and optimists for years and have found that adopting an optimistic perspective helps you become more mentally and physically resilient.

Optimism is about viewing the world from the perspective that everything that happens to you offers you an opportunity to learn more about yourself and grow as an individual. The deciding factor between an optimist and a pessimist is that the former interprets an event positively, whereas the latter will find a negative spin.

Adopting a more optimistic mindset is a proactive act of self-care that will not only increase your resilience, it will also help you to be more open and less stressed. Consequently, according to the findings of Seligman, you are healthier and far less prone to heart disease, cancer and auto-immune disorders.

Developing optimism does not necessarily need you to work with cognitive therapists. It is a habitual quality you can cultivate yourself through regular self inquiry, presence and reflection. Drawing on your own experiences, your strengths and areas you would like to improve on, you can use the art of awareness to create more empowering stories and start changing your inner dialogue over time. This chapter will show you how an optimistic perspective shapes your world from the inside out, no matter what your personal circumstances.

The next story may initially seem as though it is about many aspects of resilience, but underlying each aspect is a firm foundation of optimism. This story comes from a heart-led physician, Dr. Jill Stocker, who has learned the art of resilience by embracing the concept of 'one more time'. Her story includes personal reflections about vulnerability and creating a sense of hope and possibility in others. It also includes recommendations for practices you can incorporate into your daily life to increase your resilience and cultivate your optimism.

The Power of Possibility, and One More Time
by Jill Stocker, D.O.

What IS Resilience? Is it the ability to get up, one more time, after being knocked down for the hundredth? Is it the ability to open your heart to love, one more time, despite heartbreak after heartbreak? Is it the ability to believe in yourself, your mission, your message, your MAGIC, one more time, after countless rejections? Yes…it's ALL of those. It's about the "One More Time" factor, for me.

Is it about becoming calloused, hardened, unfeeling, and numb to thoughts, emotions, and feelings? It seems like that's what one would need to be able to do to be able to believe in the "one more time" over and over again. For self-preservation it seems only logical that one would have to become completely detached.

However… WHAT IF…you felt EVERYTHING!!! What If…you rode each wave for what it is, not knowing where it's going, until it crashed, or caressed the shore gently, then got back up and rode the next one, each wave taking you on an entirely different journey?

What if you opened your heart so incredibly wide to one word…Possibility.

What if your superpower was to wake up every morning with the childlike wonder of "Anything is possible" and such an incredible belief in yourself that you believe it can be so?

When I first began pondering my place in this book, the actual thought that came to my mind was "what story do I have to share that could possibly show resilience" (as if I wasn't resilient)? Then I realized it was all that old tape playing in the background of my mind. And the reality is, I have found my song, my music, my magic, and I DO have something to share.

For me, I have always felt that by sharing my innermost insecurities and old recordings of my mind I would be perceived as weak and die alone of my own neediness. The reality for me, though, has been, by sharing this very "perceived" weakness, it actually forges connection. Connection is our very first and basic human need and is not "needy" at all!

I've literally had people come up to me after sharing something super vulnerable, exposing my inner workings to people, and they've said "I would have never come up to you to talk to you had you not shared that". The perceptions we all have of how other people look "put together" and the "compare and despair" that follows is astonishing. It is by exposing ourselves, our "cracks" that the light is able to actually get in! Highly resilient people feel the fear and do it anyway, feel the feels and do it anyway, and expose the crack in the armor and do it anyway!

Courage is not the absence of fear, it's feeling it and doing it anyway, and perhaps even reframing and rewording the fear into excitement and possibility! When we let others know that while we may seem like we're thriving, we still have fears and self deprecating thoughts, yet we are doing it anyway, we inspire them to do the same. by knowing my mentors have felt these feels as well, it inspires me to feel them and to keep going.

Creating new neural connections in our brain actually enables us to rewire our old tape playing in the background and create new amazing music that helps us feel more alive. I used to think I wasn't very creative, when in reality, I just needed to learn how to coax out my creativity. For me, this looks like trying new things, forging new neural connections, to do so. It looks like improv classes, salsa dance classes, hot yoga, coloring, dancing and moving my body, bodysurfing and cold plunges in the ocean. The ability to try new things can literally rewire your brain.

Connecting with others and taking the risk of exposing your true self can be the scariest, and most exhilarating, freeing feeling in the world. Resilient people associate with other resilient people, because we're all on the same ladder of life. We don't judge, we help each other. Here's one crucial secret to my resilience…knowing that we're not all CRUSHING IT in all aspects of life all the time! by exposing our very humanity to others, we give others permission to do the same, and to have more self compassion for the very human nature of our being.

Acceptance is another key factor. Knowing that I am EXACTLY where I need to be on that ladder, not further ahead, but right where I am AT THAT MOMENT. The law of attraction has become quite a popular concept for people to embrace, which is great, except for one flaw. It doesn't mention the concept of expansion and contraction. The law of Acceptance for what…is…now. Quite often a mantra of mine is "Be Here Now".

Structure helps as well. Most of us have a set of personalized rituals and routines that keep us steered the right direction. Much of my life growing up was structured, followed by intense schooling/training structures. So for awhile I revolted against it, but realized that when I didn't have this structure, I didn't feel as clear and wasn't as focused with my projects. The difference is that I have developed my own set of rituals that I adhere to, rather than the ones I grew up with. I began to listen to my body, mind, and soul and what it needed the most, daily.

The majority of society, including myself originally, cares for themselves last, where really we need to put ourselves first. We can only pour from a cup that's overflowing, not from a well that's dry. We often think of only giving to other people as giving, but it's to our careers, our passions, our children, and our intimate relationships as well. Saying "Yes" to ourselves and what our body, mind, and soul needs more, and "No" to anything that doesn't nourish that is not only self care, it's self PRESERVATION, which is an actual necessity to flourish.

We get quiet, we dive deep, we aim to live in the "What IS". We listen to our body, feeding it with what it needs to process all that IS…. healthy food, people, music, dance, play, rest, sex, personal intimacy, bubble baths, massages, Netflix, and sometimes to simply lie on the floor and stare at the ceiling. Now, there's a fine line between self care and isolation, and it's important to understand the distinction. Introspection is a powerful, scary, and sometimes lonely, act. But the more we can be observers of our thoughts, feelings, emotions, behaviors, rather than judges of them, the more we can learn and grow from them.

Self knowledge is a superpower that few dare to explore. Self acceptance and self compassion are even more difficult. Self discipline and self cheerleading are game changers. A vision without a plan is just a dream. by learning what motivates us, what fills our hearts, and what sets our soul and entire body on fire, as well as what terrifies us, what are our innermost repeated self sabotaging dialogues, we align ourselves with endless possibilities. We look for the lesson, the "opportunity for growth" in everything. We look at things that happen that may at first appear as obstacles, as mere re-directions. And reframe the question "Why is this happening TO me?" to "Why is this happening FOR me?".

Our greatest joy, agony, and FREEDOM, is knowing ourselves, deeply, intimately, sacredly. For it is in knowing ourselves that we can then be able to relate in a more compassionate, loving way with others. I often think perhaps I was given certain challenges to first work through myself, to then be able to share with and show others how and to mirror new ways for them.

I used to think self reliance was the way....NO!!! That leads to isolation, the exact opposite of connection. Where and when did we get he notion that we have to do everything ourselves? For me, and many of us, it's modeling of our ancestors (parents, grandparents, etc.) My grandparents grew up in the Great Depression. They were extremely hard workers and savers, and if there was a job to be done, they did it themselves. This was a great work ethic to learn from for sure, but just as I speak to my patients about themselves and their children, life lessons are just as important as, and sometimes more important than, school lessons.

As a physician, I can honestly say I've learned more from my life lessons than my school training…for myself, and for my patients, and for the generations to come (my children). I am "re"modeling for my patients, giving them permission to live all aspects of their lives. This is something I'm also modeling for my children. Life is not about how much money or things you have, but the experience and rapture of feeling alive, yet so much of our self worth and measure of "success" is often tied up in things and status.

I used to do EVERYTHING….work full time, seeing sometimes forty patients a day, pick up the kids from daycare, cook dinner, take the kids to soccer and ballet, then picnics/parks/lemonade stands on the weekends, interspersing cleaning the house and doing the laundry throughout all of that. Yet I found myself not ENJOYING any part of it, not even the stuff that was "supposed to" be fun! I wasn't fully present for any of it. I didn't get my hair wet or jump on the trampoline with my kids…I WATCHED and DID, but wasn't BEING or LIVING.

I realized that my kids would only be little once, and at that point I employed help, a housekeeper. Because I had grown up with seeing my mom do everything too, I thought this was something I needed to do as well, and had initial shame about needing help. The tradeoff though was that I started to feel like I could breathe, and I started to wake up to my life and feel alive!

There seems to be a societal stigma that women/mothers should be the "nurturers" and do everything in the home, and I think it's possible to be a nurturing mother while also providing an example of being anything you want to be. Now, I live life to the fullest and get my hair wet, body surf with my kids, and GIGGLE!! My kids all take bubble baths on their own as part of their self care, and my daughter just spoke at the inaugural Global Luminary Activation Experience. Me turning over the care of my house to someone else enabled me to be more present for myself and my children to help lead them and myself down a more connected and fulfilling path

by employing help, in whatever area of life we need, it enables to be fully present for what IS. Ditch the guilt of what things are "supposed to" look like. Pain is inevitable (in life, in relationships, in growth), but suffering is optional. So rather than being uncomfortable in what your life is right now if you're not where you want to be, try something different that's uncomfortable, like bodysurfing, or painting, or co-author a book, and see what happens with the brain rewiring.

This doesn't just mean delegating tasks to others, but also not keeping all those feelings, thoughts to yourself to figure out and handle. Again, self reliance leads to isolation, the opposite of connection. It's connection that helps us mirror new experiences and thought patterns. Being uncomfortable in the unknown rather than knowing what's next or being able to fit everything into a neat bento box of emotions/feelings/thoughts. by sharing with someone else, it helps us realize we're not alone on this amazing, and sometimes terrifying journey called life. It helps us realize our common humanity in one another. It's time we break down the tall walls we have built, and instead create a patchwork quilt of ourselves that tells a wildly unique story and can take us to the next level of the most amazing magic carpet ride ever. Asking for help is humbling, and connecting, remember that.

An attitude of gratitude begets more things to be grateful for, as well as more heart warming emotions. All emotions are welcome, there aren't really "good" or "bad" emotions, they're all just messengers and can bring us useful information. Having recently been part of a live demonstration of Heart Math, I could visibly see the effects of something that I had been practicing for years, as well as confirm a new habit I had created for myself. The mere thought of something unpleasant created an excitatory/agitated reaction in my heart, not even feeling the feelings associated with the thought. Therefore, the more of those thoughts I allow, the more of those detrimental effects on my heart. The opposite was true as well.

by merely looking at something I was grateful for, my heart rate automatically slowed and relaxed, without even feeling the physical feelings of gratitude. Therefore, the gratitude list I've been writing every morning for years has been serving to fill my heart with even more love, which I believe allows for the "one more time" and "possibility" of my mornings to unfold. For many, when they think of things they're grateful for, they think of tangible things. But it's seeing ALL of it....the love of my children, my health that keeps me remain active and able to help others, the magic inside me that inspires others.

This leads me to the last thing that I believe to be of utmost importance to being resilient....my purpose. For so long I knew I wanted to be a doctor, which I became. But it wasn't until the past few years that I have truly found my purpose in life, in all of humanity (yes, the sky's the limit once you start allowing it!). Once you discover you have a greater purpose on this planet, waking up with wonder and possibility every morning becomes more the norm than not. It's okay if you don't quite know it, as most of us are on a hamster wheel of life just doing rather than being and exploring what lights us up. Once you feel the inner rumbling, follow it, explore it.

Your purpose can evolve, it will evolve, because you will too. If you don't quite know what yours is right now, or even believe you have one, I'm telling you I believe in you. And I believe you are here for a purpose, and the magical unfolding of it has only just begun with you reading this.

To recap, when you can't quite see any light......please remember this:

One more time...always

Embrace Possibility

Connection

Self care and self success rituals

Self reliance leads to self sabotage, asking for help isn't weak, it forges connection!

An attitude of gratitude can literally rewire your heart and brain, it all starts with one thought

Remember to BE where you are, at all times, each part is integral to your entire journey and trajectory.

You're exactly ON TIME where ever you are in your journey, sit with that.

About the Author

Dr. Jill Stocker is an expert in Age Management Medicine and Hormonal Optimization. Her unique expertise and personal experience imparts a special dimension for promoting optimum, whole-body/mind/spirit wellness by combining her medical expertise, along with personal and intuitive experiences to guide people to the best version of themselves.

She has made it her life's work to help women and men *Reclaim Their Juiciness*... physically, mentally, emotionally, spiritually, and sexually. It's about CELEBRATING, not medicating; and going from surviving to THRIVING! Part of Jill's mission is to empower people to demand more from their healers, reinforcing you are more than just a lab number, and to also educate healers on the importance of Listening to Listen, not to diagnose.

Dr. Jill

www.jillstocker.com

Tips to optimize your optimism

You can guarantee that no one but you will fully recognize your own abilities.

Think about all the times you overcame obstacles without telling anyone, or you mastered your inner critic even though it was working hard to trip you up. How would it feel to start more consciously noticing these things, so that you can inwardly celebrate yourself?

The more you celebrate your wins, the more optimistic you will feel about your ability to overcome challenging circumstances in your life. Start telling yourself about all the times you succeeded when you least expected it so that you build your optimism from within.

Remind yourself regularly of the times when you were able to calm yourself down or control your mind in some way. This will help you to be more optimistic about your ability to repeat this another time. Remember no one will champion you the way you can, so become your own champion!

When you are optimistic about life and your ability to create your future, remember that your mind starts looking for evidence to substantiate your beliefs, which builds your resilience.

Cast your mind to a time when you emerged triumphant from a situation that you found fearful. What positive lessons about yourself can you take away from this? How will you remember these? Could you find three words that encapsulate this?

The clearer you become on your uniques strengths and qualities, the easier you will find it to adopt an optimistic viewpoint rather than a pessimistic one.

To boost your sense of optimism from a worldview perspective, seek out positive news stories and websites who are focussed on making the world a better place. Examples are The Good News Network www.goodnewsnetwork.org and the Happy News by Emily Coxhead www.thehappynewspaper.com

Limit your intake of negative news and get better at noticing what inputs make you feel negative or send you into a downward spiral of worrying about the future. You can still stay in touch with what is happening in the world without watching the news every day, reading newspapers or scrolling on social media, so feed your brain in a conscious way and look after your happy hormones!

To end your day, it is well worth setting aside a few minutes to write down three wins for the day and reflect on what aspects of your character contributed to them going well. Make these wins as small or large as you like and when you write them down using pen and paper, it stimulates your Reticular Activating System, the portal that filters important information going into your brain.

This may seem like a very small gesture, but when you repeat it often enough, you will be surprised by how this improves your quality of life.

Your life does not change in big sweeping gestures, or dramatic interludes. It is the small intentional actions you take regularly that create change and momentum, and ultimately improve each day.

Resilience Trait #6
Confidence

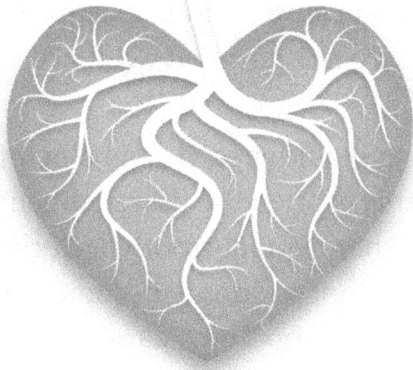

The word confidence comes from the Latin word fidere', which means to trust. Confidere literally translates as 'with trust'; therefore having self-confidence means you have trust in yourself.

Those who are confident have trust in their ability to emerge intact from life's challenges, which gives them a sense of self-assurance, grounding and inner calm. Confident people show up more authentically, are self-reliant and more likely to keep going when others might give up. As a result, their confidence often acts like a self-fulfilling prophecy as they succeed in areas where less confident people fail as a result of giving up sooner.

Like every resilience trait, confidence is not an innate or fixed characteristic. It can be cultivated by anyone and improved upon over time. Confidence is all about believing in yourself, so the starting point is to start believing you can build confidence, no matter what evidence you feel you have to the contrary!

When building confidence, it can be helpful to address anxiety first, as this is often the dominant emotion that arises in any situation where you currently lack confidence. Resilient people do not suddenly become fearless or immune to nervousness or anxiety. They learn how to manage themselves better when these feelings arise, so that they stay calm in challenging circumstances and develop greater trust in themselves.

Anxiety and worry arise from the part of our nervous system that wants to keep us safe, which means that they are often accompanied by physiological symptoms such as shakiness, upset stomach, insomnia and low mood. Add to this chaotic thinking and unhealthy compensation methods and it is easy to see how this can drain your sense of self-trust and confidence.

Learning how to create calm for yourself addresses the physiological responses in your system so that you can breathe more fully, think more clearly and open your mind up to receive new insights. Studies show that regular practice of meditation, whether focusing on the breath, a mantra or an object of visualization can help dissipate anxious energy.

This physiological shift increases your ability to problem-solve effectively, giving you a stronger sense of security and belief in your own capabilities. In addition to this, developing the skill of focused concentration can help you block out habitual negative self-talk, restoring harmony to your body and brain.

The more adept you become at managing your state, the easier it becomes to start imagining yourself handling challenging situations in a more positive way. The practice of regularly visualizing yourself acting with more confidence in specific settings, is a valuable tool to adopt when it comes to building your confidence. It may seem like make-believe, but neuroscientists have proven through brain-imaging studies that subconscious pathways in your brain activate when you visualize specific outcomes. This means you can retrain your brain to believe you are more confident and you can open your mind to new positive possibilities.

Building confidence is yet another self-fulfilling prophecy, as the more you prove to yourself that you can handle new situations, the more confident in yourself you become. Understanding that feelings of anxiety are physiological responses very similar to excitement also means that you can train yourself to reframe the feelings, so that when they arise, you can let go of the automatic anxiety that drains you and instead tell yourself you feel excited.

To increase your ability to trust in yourself, you can access several free guided meditations on my website or on iTunes that will help train you to be calm and confident when you need to be.

You can also learn to calm yourself with deep breathing, practicing yoga, exercising, or meditation. Shifting your state by getting out in nature, listening to music, doing something creative and connecting with others can also help.

Our next story, by Malin Hedlund, proves that adding several of these confidence boosting activities to your daily routine, and creating your own rituals to bring peaceful calm into your life, can do wonders when life becomes overwhelming or stressful. Her story demonstrates that we can return to our cool, calm and resourceful state even while the world is crumbling around us. Malin faced one of the biggest challenges a parent could face, moving across the world as her young adult children made moves of their own. And she shares with us the shaky emotions that went with the decision making process, while she dealt with the nervous feeling of not knowing how her business would evolve after moving to another country. Malin outlines a process that she used for herself, and teaches her clients that will help you, too, create the life of your dreams, even when one dream is ending.

And the final story in this chapter, by Catherine McLeod, highlights just how easy it is to lose our confidence when the outside world sends us bullies and doubters. Fortunately, even when our confidence has been diminished by forces outside of us, we can always tap back into it — via our intuition and spiritual guidance — to return to our natural state of power and peace.

CREATE Your Dream Life
by Malin Hedlund

The beginning of the year started out great. I was energetic, enthusiastic and had set up amazing goals and intentions for the year. I knew what I wanted to accomplish. No excuses, it was time to get cracking.

I quickly found that nothing seemed to be working. After nearly every business meeting, I got positive feedback and the clients seemed happy. But I often ended up getting a "no" which sounded like "we will keep in touch", "maybe next year", or "let's meet again after the holidays."

During this time, I started thinking about doing something else, or at least changing my focus to my Swedish clients. Uncertainty and doubt about my capabilities found their way through my thoughts, which I did not want to admit. I watched how others worked, what their strategies and requirements were, what type of marketing they practiced. by taking bits and pieces from what I saw others do, I thought I had figured out a new approach to use. It ended up feeling more forced than fun. Having fun at work is a priority of mine as it makes work so much easier!

At home things were also uncertain. We did not know whether we would be staying in the Netherlands, or whether it was time to move somewhere else. My positive mindset kept me thinking that it does not matter where in the world I live because my job can be done anywhere. Therefore, I did not care too much about the subject, and instead put all my focus into work. My single-focus on work led me to doing workshops for free to show what I was capable of, but also the occasional paid job. Yet, it did not seem to work.

Meanwhile during this period my father had fallen ill with cancer and was in a poor state. My dear father who is stronger and healthier than most elderly! It felt so unfair. My father's situation was constantly on my mind and worried me sick. "Will he be okay; how long until he's good again; how is my mother doing; how do my kids feel about it; why don't I live in the same country as my parents?"

I flew home to Sweden to take care of my mother, to support her and keep her company while my father was in the hospital. And of course to visit my father and to keep him happy. He had gotten so tiny -- it was as if the cancer had eaten him. "How could he possibly regain his strength?" I kept thinking. Especially with the awful food he was getting in the hospital.

He kept fighting. He was determined that this was not the end. I helped him with his nutrition and exercise program. It was amazing to see the amount of work he put into his physical and mental wellbeing, with my supportive mother right by his side. My parents are true role models in how to love and care for each other NO MATTER WHAT.

Back to (another) reality

Suddenly, we were on the move; we just did not know where. Could be Dubai, could be Sweden… nobody knew. While my husband and I were waiting for some sort of verdict, the movers were busy packing our stuff. The strange feeling of knowing that you had to move out but had no idea where you would move in was frightening. No person in their right mind would ever put themselves under this type of pressure. No mother would willingly put their kids through this. But I knew my two children were happy, so I did not feel like the most terrible mother after all.

Meditation, journaling and reading became very important to my wellbeing during this time to help me cope with the uncertainty, anxiety and nervousness, and to be there for my family. It was challenging at times, but it worked. Finally, we made the unexpected decision to stay in the Netherlands!

A fresh start

I soon notice that my business is booming and everything is running smoothly. But I do not see what I am doing differently. The only difference I do sense is internal, in my body, heart and mind. I have finally achieved a sense of peace and tranquillity. The connection between my wellbeing and the success of my business is undeniable. Through all the ups and downs I have kept my vision as an adviser, reminded myself of why I want to help people develop and become the best version of themselves. Sure, at times I may have pondered whether this really was my destiny in life, whether I really did love my job. But deep down I knew that this is what I wanted to do. I am meant to make a difference in the world by contributing to peoples' wellbeing, power, happiness and fulfillment.

Staying in the Netherlands was a good decision because I could continue with my business as usual. Working with renowned, global companies made me realize that I was living my dream; working with the best clients who always put a smile on myself and make me feel valuable!

My excitement only lasted for a little while, however, as my husband soon came home and told me he had gotten a job opportunity in the US. He would finally be able to realize HIS dream. I was stunned. I could not find any words. When we decided to stay at least four more years in the Netherlands, I made a solid plan on how to grow my business, and now he came with this idea? Instead of telling him my initial feelings I started throwing questions at him – why, what makes this a better option than staying, how come you changed your mind, are you sure this is what we need right now, is this really the best approach, etc.

Despite knowing how thrilled my husband was about this new opportunity, all I felt was anger, frustration, and disappointment. What about me? My dreams? And my vision? I always tell my clients to go after their dreams, yet this time I felt very uncertain whether it was the right choice. I felt left behind, forgotten, cheated on. But who was I to stop my husband from achieving his dream of living in the USA? His American dream.

More challenges?!

Working on my patience, emotions, thoughts and temper is difficult when all I really want is to stay where we are and keep living the life we currently live. Interactions with my husband often end with me being irritated. It feels like a huge uphill battle to tackle this new chapter in our lives. Thinking about all our to-do's, all the planning, all the arrangements that need to happen before the move make me exhausted. Finding a real estate agent for the house, SELLING the house (which we just finished renovating), choosing a moving company, applying for Visas and getting accepted, the list goes on. One of the most difficult battles I struggle with is leaving friends whom we have established amazing friendships with. But the biggest question looming over my head is "what in the world am I going to do about my entrepreneurship once we move?" I refuse to give up all the hard work I have put into my company.

It took dozens of discussions with different experts and even more sleepless nights because I was so determined to make this work. My company will continue because I have a VISION and big DREAMS but making it work requires all my energy, focus, and willingness, which I feel like I am running out of. My head was like a dryer on full speed, and it did not seem to end. I wanted to scream: STOP, please give me answers, peace and rest.

Although my business is very dear to my heart, my children lie closer. Being away from them makes moving across the Atlantic even more strenuous than finding a solution for my business. My 21-year-old already lives on her own in the Netherlands, so I have gotten used to not seeing her every day anymore. My son, who just turned 17, decided he does not want to move with us to the USA. He is determined that moving back to Sweden is the right choice for him, despite having two years left of high school. His dreams about playing soccer on a professional level is strongly connected to that.

Although I had never imagined my kids moving out (almost) at the same time, the coach within me says that this is the right solution. After years of teaching and preaching the importance of following your dreams, doing what you love, and daring to step out of your comfort zone, I am now facing an emotional roller coaster following my son's decision. Motherhood still means making sure he is safe, loved, taken care of, that he has food, shelter, comfort, and that he finishes his primary education!! But that does not mean my son has to live at home…does it?

I was not mentally prepared for such a big change, but my son undoubtedly was. He thought through ALL possible scenarios and is convinced that nothing can stop him. Being so far from my children, is that what I stand for? NO, it is not but my children have made up their minds about their future and I am no one to stop it. They are adults, or at least becoming adults and shape their own lives according to their dreams and wishes.

So, my husband and I allowed my son to make this big move, in fact, we praise him and admire him for being so brave. Yet, it is difficult knowing I will not be close to my children – it hurts, it makes me sad, it makes my heart ache. Friends admire us and tell us to be proud of our courageous children, saying they will be absolutely fine! "You have done an excellent job as a parent" they say. I want to believe that this is true, so I rest my case.

How to CREATE the life you dream of

It is easy to criticize yourself, to look for flaws, judge yourself and your decisions. Such behaviour leads to a negative spiral, and the more flaws we look for in ourselves, the more we find. A negative attitude and outlook on problems become the result of this negative spiral. Thereafter it becomes increasingly difficult to find creative solutions.

We are so much better off giving ourselves love, positive feelings, and support. And it is important to tell ourselves that we are SMART and fully capable of making good decisions. Thus, I decide to trust my intuition and my decisions.

You have probably heard the saying: "When life gives you lemons, make lemonade". But how do you do that?! How do you create a nice, harmonious environment when life gives you a lemon? Below, you will find a method I use to guide my clients in such a situation, and in this case, the method I use to guide myself.

C CLARITY: create a vision and direction for your life

R RITUALS: reflections, self-awareness

E EXPAND: your potential, step out of your comfort zone

A ATTITUDE: mindset and habits, ways of approaching situations

T TAKE ACTION: small steps are important, a vision without action won't lead anywhere

E EVALUATE: what's working? What's not working?

The big move

During this tough period, I intensify my meditation frequency. I keep to my rituals, make sure I have time for myself and my wellbeing. When we get to the climax, the hardest part of the process, I meditate several times a day, in silence, with music or with guidance, always in stillness to keep me grounded. Walks in nature also give me peace and tranquillity. I practice more yoga. These little moments of self-care and awareness are vital to my sanity during stressful times. That is something I have learnt from past mistakes.

When you think you do not have time to work out, do yoga, meditate, etc., that is when you need it the most! It is so easy to think you need to focus on your 'to-do list', but in reality your priority should be your mental and physical wellbeing. Before ANYTHING else.

My CREATE system includes guidance for each step. The very first step in changing something about your life is asking yourself what and how you want it. You must be one hundred percent certain, or CLEAR about what is important and why. When you have a direction to follow, a VISION, you can just plug in your mental 'GPS' and thereafter follow the path. If you do not know what you want your life to be like there is a big risk you will be living someone else's life.

The next step in CREATE is RITUALS. Rituals are well thought-through (mindful) actions, which adjust to and support one's VISION. Essentially the things that need to happen daily to get closer to your VISION. It is all about making lasting, powerful strategies that ensure you are going in the right direction.

Another important decision I made was to get a mentor. Somebody who helps me out, guides me, pushes me, and sees parts of me that I am not able to see. Often times we think we are getting out of our comfort zone, but in reality, we handle things just like we always do. Nothing new here. This is when we get to step 3 in the model: EXPAND your comfort zone.

I ponder whether it is smart to get a coach when I am so out of balance. Am I ready to work on myself? When is the best time to get a coach? With the experience I now have, I strongly recommend getting a coach when you NEED one – not when you think you are 'ready' to get one. It is incredibly valuable to be able to talk to somebody, even if you think you can handle it on your own. A coach will often ask you questions you have never thought about before, or make you see your problems in a different light. A coach can help you overcome your worries and fears and push you to step out of your comfort zone, even more than you would yourself.

I am tired, I cry easily, I am anxious about what is to come. The only place where I can fully disconnect from all the move-related stress is at work. At work, I focus solely on my clients, put myself in their shoes, am completely mindful during these situations, this is where I find an energy boost because I love helping people and seeing progress!

Work affects my ATTITUDE, which is step 4 in the CREATE model, and my mindset about everything else. If you look up the word attitude in the dictionary, it says that it is "a settled way of thinking of feeling about something". However, I firmly believe that you have the full capacity to choose your attitude and the ways in which you respond to things happening around you. It is not easy, but it is simple.

The toughest part is not deciding but TAKING ACTION. This is the 5th step in the process and means that any little action you manage to do is better than nothing. Wow, how hard I have worked to change my attitude. There are days when I feel like nothing matters anymore because I am not in control, but then I give myself a little pep-talk and tell myself that it is better to see everything that IS going my way, what works and so on, and thereby become stronger and more focused. Little "ant-steps" at a time, as I like to say. When we take these small steps we increase our self-confidence, which gives us motivation to keep going. My motivation in this messy situation is getting the honor to work with wonderful people. People who have a vision or goal in mind, but who do not know exactly how to achieve it.

The biggest change in myself is that I accept who I am and what I am capable of, which results in a more relaxed, easy-going attitude towards work and clients. I no longer have the energy to adapt to what I think my clients expect from me, but instead start with the intention of helping them reach their dreams and goals using my best ability. This turns out to be a successful method as I get more and more requests, and eventually end up getting my biggest business-deal so far! To me, it is very clear that this change has happened because of my change in attitude. I am only seeing this change now, a while after it happened. This is the last step in the process: EVALUATE. It is important to make a summary or evaluation of what has happened and why, as well as how it could be approached differently next time from what you have learned.

It is vital to remember that there is always a way if we are open to change something about ourselves or our lives. Even though you may think there is no way for you to achieve your dreams because of age, money, etc., there is ALWAYS a way. You just have to be willing to work hard, be prepared to step on unfamiliar territory, and work your 'mental muscles'. If you follow this equation, nothing can stop you. All you have to do is C R E A T E your own reality.

About the Author

Malin Hedlund is the founder and owner of MH Leadership. With more than twenty years of experience in creating and delivering leadership programs for companies of all sizes, she empowers ambitious female leaders/entrepreneurs to flourish by inspiring them to find their unique flow through prioritizing their own wellbeing. Her expertise takes a holistic approach, driving success in others through a combination of individual coaching and team coaching while promoting a healthy, active lifestyle. Malin has multiple years of international experience, she's also a certified Personal Fitness Trainer.

Find out more about Malin Hedlund at

https://www.mhleadership.com/

https://www.linkedin.com/in/malinhedlund/

https://www.facebook.com/MHLeadership/

Reclaiming My Intuition
by Catherine McLeod

When I was young I was fearless!! When our family bought a parachute to fly us above our speed boat I was the first to try it. I 100% trusted my intuition, felt comforted by the spirits that visited and spent time with me, and I loved life to its absolute fullest. When a spirit moose visited me in my bedroom I didn't think it was strange, it felt completely normal to me and when it licked my hand I was exhilarated!!

The spirit world has always been there for me and I have always trusted and loved the guidance received from my 'team'. But as I got older and spoke to people about what I saw and heard, I felt like a freak. So much so that in my early 20's I turned off this wonderful gift, as I wanted to be accepted and not have people look at me like I was from another planet.

This conscious decision to turn off my gift to communicate with the spirit world, and to listen to and trust my intuition led to me being surrounded by people who didn't have my best interests at heart. I ended up in a career that I am grateful for, but is not where my purpose lies.

When I turned off my gift I essentially set myself adrift. I cut the cord that kept my soul attached to the spirit world and let myself loose like a boat on the water to follow the flow and land where it may. Where it landed me was on the other side of the country in a crazy busy job that eventually burnt me out.

I had worked as a caregiver for aged clients for 13 years before I graduated as a Registered Nurse. I absolutely loved my graduate year in plastic surgery, and the Emergency department of a very busy city hospital, but my heart remained in aged care. So after a 12 month graduate program I found myself back in aged care working in a residential facility as a Registered Nurse. Oh my, how I loved this job. This role was the most rewarding one I had ever had, and I really felt like I could make a difference in people's lives. Being with a person and assisting them to live their best life until their end of days is a role that I feel is a privilege and must not be taken lightly. Throughout this role I made some very valuable friendships, mentored and taught a lot of junior staff, and thoroughly enjoyed every minute. But at the same time I felt that I had more to offer.

It was at this time that I felt the pull to go home. I had lived away from home for many years travelling all over the east coast of Australia, the UK and western Australia. My gorgeous mum let me know of a role that was being advertised which was the next step up in my career and I thought I had no chance of getting it, but I applied, and much to my surprise I got the job!! The role was that of a deputy director of nursing in a large aged care facility and as I didn't think I would get the job, I felt that I had to live up to high expectations. So naturally I worked really hard learning the role and what was expected of me. After 6 months the facility manager resigned and I landed myself in that role first by default and then on purpose, as I eventually applied for the role. BIG MISTAKE!!

My intuition was yelling at me that this wasn't the right path to go down but I ignored it as it seemed like a logical progression of my career. Who would turn down an opportunity like this? It would be crazy and I felt that I would be looked down upon by my family or that I would let them down if I turned it down. Silly really, but that is how I felt at the time.

With that in mind I threw myself into this new role. I worked very long hours, answered emails and phone calls from colleagues and bosses at all hours of the evening as I believed this made me a good, dedicated employee. This then became an expectation. At one point I was doing the roles of 4 people, including working the floor on the night shift when the RN called in sick, but the emails, calls and expectations did not let up. One night following a night shift I had worked to fill in for the RN, my boss emailed me with jobs I needed to complete prior to 10am the next day. I had already worked a full day shift plus a night shift and was exhausted, but such was the expectation.

It got to the point where I thought I could not go on. I was being bullied by other people in the organisation, my blood pressure was very high, so high I was at risk of having a stroke, my anxiety levels were through the roof and I was living off of adrenaline. After one night shift a colleague came to me very upset and was crying, I held her and let her cry and debrief. During this my entire team that I was to handover to ignored us, walked on in and watched us. I was repulsed and disgusted. How could adults not understand privacy and let another person cry and debrief without

221

walking in and just stare until I huddled her out of the room to give hand over? It was after this particular handover that after everyone had left my office, I closed the door, leaned against it, slid to the floor and sobbed by heart out. I stayed there for about 20 minutes and let it all out.

While I was on the floor, I had a moment. I saw myself from the outside in, it was like I left my body and was looking down on myself at the person that I had become. I didn't like what I saw. It was the wake up call I needed. During this out of body experience I remembered the spirits, my intuition and guide team and wondered how I had become this blubbering mess on the floor.

I made a decision that day to turn my gift back on and I quit my job.

Following this bold decision I had a small moment of complete and utter panic. As I sat at my computer writing my resignation letter my mind wandered and it is here that the panic set in. What was I doing??!! I was in a well paying job and was throwing it all away with no other job to go to and a child to support…argh!!! Then I made a decision to lean into this feeling and it was at this time I felt complete and utter warmth come over me and I knew right away that I was going to be ok. I knew that my guide team were with me as that same feeling of warmth and inner knowing was very familiar. It was the same feeling I used to feel when I was younger. So with that I finished writing my resignation letter, hit the send button, and never looked back.

Now although I never looked back, the feeling of total exhaustion, emotional instability, anxiety and feelings of worthlessness remained with me. I was burnt out. Anyone who is a parent knows how challenging it can be raising another human being even without our own stuff to deal with. Being a single parent comes with even more challenges. My biggest concern at this point was that I was failing as a parent and was not being the role model I wanted to be for my daughter. And it was here that my road to recovery from burnout began.

Recovering from burnout, for me, has been a journey of self discovery. I've rediscovered the joy of spirit, of listening to and following my intuition and trusting that everything will be ok.

This process of trusting my intuition led me to all things woo woo. I know how that sounds but my life needed a complete overhaul and what better way to do this than to do the opposite of what I had been doing. I began by completing a Tarot course which then turned into a weekly gathering of women who supported and loved each other unconditionally. I am grateful that these women are still in my life today as they helped me see that it is ok to be a little different and it is ok to let others in and allow myself to trust again. With these women we went to shamanic sweat lodges, we made medicine drums, we learnt to laugh and listen to nature and we bonded as a sisterhood. These women showed me that being a strong, sensitive and intuitive woman is ok, they led me back to my femininity.

This journey eventually led me to Reiki. It was always on my radar when I was younger but I felt like it was some weird thing that other, more enlightened people did. When it came up again in my dreams and in my intuition I decided to trust and follow my intuition and I am so grateful that I did because Reiki has changed my life!! It's so funny how life or the universe seems to provide you with just what you need right at the time you need it. This is how I found my Reiki Master. She popped up in my news feed on Facebook the same week that I had had the dream about Reiki and when I closed my eyes and leant into this, asking my guide team if this was the best decision for my highest good, I got a resounding Yes!! It also felt right within my gut.

The next logical step was to schedule time with her to begin my Reiki journey and as it turned out, start on my path to further self discovery. I booked in with her to learn Reiki Level 1 and it was this meeting that changed everything. Completing this level and the consequent levels after this to become a Reiki Master, deepened my connection to source energy and myself.

The relationship within myself has always been a tumultuous one. As a young person I had a definite sense of self, I knew exactly who I was and no one was going to tell me otherwise. Then life happened. I had my heart broken a couple of times, then became burnt out in that job and all of this made me second guess myself and I was constantly asking "who am I"? Initially I looked outside of myself for the answer to this question. Then I looked to others, people around me, to see who I was. I never actually asked them the question but I looked at their character, at who THEY were to discover who I was. I did this because I have come to learn that what and who we attract into our lives is a direct reflection of what we are putting out into the universe and what is going on within ourselves.

Doing this on a daily basis was quite honestly exhausting at first but oh so necessary as it gave me great insight into who I was. I say was because throughout this process of going within after looking outside of myself caused me to change who I was and start living my life on purpose. If someone or something triggered a less than positive reaction or feeling for me this was and still is a wonderful indicator that I have something within myself to work through and release. Doing energy work is how I work though these things and release them. It is amazing what comes up when I do a healing on myself, sometimes it is something from a past life or an old wound or trauma that I had blocked out and needed a gentle reminder to consciously bring it back into awareness in order to release it. Of course there are times when I can not do this on my own so through the process of clearing and learning to trust others again, I ask for help. Sometimes this help is via a medical professional but if it is energy work that I need assistance with I ask one of my two mentors and my Reiki Master.

Working with energy has been the most rewarding way for me to recover from burnout. It has allowed me to understand that when I put my trust in someone to work with my energy I am trusting them to love me unconditionally, as working with another person's energy is one of the most intimate things we can do. There is nowhere to hide as our energy speaks a different language and it shows us what is for our highest good. When I work with clients I am humbled that they have placed their trust in me. This work is the most beautiful work I have ever done. Energy medicine has opened me up to new and fulfilling friendships, which I believe will last a lifetime.

As you can see I am quite passionate about Reiki and energy work so of course when I began my Reiki journey in Level 1 I could not just leave it at that. I am now a Reiki Master, Angelic Reiki Practitioner (soon to be Master Teacher), Sound healer and Intuitive healer. Learning how to navigate energy and the emotional causes, among other things, that can upset our energies has been my greatest healing experience. It has taught me to really look inside myself, to metaphorically turn over every rock, walk down every inner stream and discover who I really am and what makes me tick. It has also led me to believe in myself and my abilities more than I ever thought possible. My connection to spirit is incredible.

My journey is far from over as I believe we learn something new everyday, be that new knowledge about ourselves or new knowledge about the universe and the world we live in. My days now are spent enjoying the moment, not sweating the small stuff and helping others on their journey. I love learning new things and meeting new people and am happy to say that I am now free from burnout. I believe that learning about energy and Reiki has allowed me to become resilient. Now when things in my life are challenging I use my intuition to look within myself and learn what it is I need to let go and Reiki is a tool that assists me in this process.

My goal is to continue to inspire myself and others to live their best life, continue to practise and teach energy medicine and trust that my intuition always has my best interest at heart.

About the Author

Catherine is an 8th generation Usui Reiki Master, Angelic Reiki Practitioner, Lightworker Activator, Master Portal Navigator and lover of all things energy. Catherine's mission is to assist women to clear what blocks them from moving forward and stepping into who they are truly meant to be -- an Intrepid Warrior Woman.

Connect with Catherine Online:

www.xionspiritualhealing.com

www.facebook.com/xionspiritualhealing

www.instagram.com/xion.spiritual.healing/

Triumph of Love in Life
by Alexsa Covelli

The power of resilience doesn't come on a wave of inspiration, like in the movies. It starts resonating from the moment of conception with the insistence of a heartbeat moving towards the moment we take our first breath. The most integral part of us as kinetic, spiritual, and intellectual beings is our adaptation process, formed by our inherent design, developed by choice into empowerment.

I believe with every fiber of my being; We are born to overcome anything into the life we were made to love. We are lovable in our essence. Most people believe everything is the same energy consciousness; I hold a different truth. I see life created in a sovereign order with unique clarification where every breath is one-of-a-kind.

Infinite possibilities culminate into a spectrum of choice balanced with learning consequences. We are all here to learn, that is the gift of existence. The purpose of consciousness is to learn reality versus delusion, and excellence from inferior dysfunction, most notably to put right from wrong in the context which is best for you.

I learned this the hard way as a young orphan, with a host of challenges as my inheritance was squandered by foster people, and I endured unspeakable abuse of all kinds. I was always afraid since my very existence seemed to cause a resentment I didn't understand. When you are alone, without family, predators are aplenty. There were also challenges with an educational system that punished me for my intelligence and ambidextrous ability.

I grew up in a time where adults were trying to find themselves in every place except their skin. It was one of the worst generations of parenting or caregiving, from my point of view. Society had moved away from keeping children safe and family a priority as a means to a fast-paced end.

To claim our birthright, we have to hone into our perpetual, versatile strength of attainment. We must force our focus to the greater good of our soul in physical form. The soul isn't superior to the body; in my opinion, it's another reflection of the essence in empathy with nature. It's the spirit with cells, numbered, calculated, measured, and weighed for a perfect effect.

Therefore, the aspects of our conditioning responses that form our admirable traits are from our body in a soul reflection. I realize that resilience isn't just a mental attitude to program in your day. It's not a jolt of inspiration that lifts you in hard times.

A time of terror

I endured sixteen years of terror, targeted by a psychopathic stalker who kept me in perpetual fear of the next traumatic event. Those times were extreme experiences that could never go in a book in case my children should see it. The last time I would ever be beaten by him was after I walked into a police station to get a restraining order.

I finally decided I would do what everyone claims a domestic violence victim should do. My intuition told me not to go, but I thought I was weak. I had heard someone talking about someone who was being abused as if they were trash because they "let them get away with it." It was a mistake of infinite proportions to walk into that station.

Afterward, before I even got out of my car, the stalker's hand was on my neck. Prior to this day he said he took it easy on me, but I didn't believe him. Then my ribs knew pain like never before. Laying outside my home, apparently lifeless, he thought he finally had accomplished killing me, so he sent someone to pick up the body. I wasn't on the rocks of my driveway. I had crawled through leaves and grass, barely conscious, up the stairs to my porch.

I could have let the pain echoing from every part of me be the only thing I noticed. For a few minutes, I forgot I had a child depending on me and thought I it was my time to die. The haze of agony seemed so easy to slip away; it could have been my last breath.

Instead, I saw the inner strength to realize my purpose. It was the song of my cells, a forward-driving momentum. I heard it coming from inside of me. Waling at times, and at others a banshee cry in the love famished desert, I listened to myself despite all the other noise which said I was unworthy, ugly, shouldn't have been born, a burden, on and on. Broken and bleeding, I felt my day of triumph resounding in opportunity. "NO, I've got to live. I must live through this!"

My soul's heartbeat felt another call, another truth to believe in, which sought to empower me. The biology of our being does speak to us in secret places between our beliefs and perceptions. It echoes that we are resilient in this moment, urging us to remain steadfast towards our goals. We matter because we come from love and we live purposefully in our every role.

My daughter mattered. I had still not been loved or appreciated as a wife in an epic love story relationship. So I couldn't give up, although breathing was excruciating. Indeed when every breath hurt, it is very traumatic to live through, and I did it without drugs or help. I managed by a miracle of life force to make it to my bed. My young daughter bandaged my lungs with a towel. I stuck a rag between my legs because I couldn't go to the bathroom.

I had a concussion. As I lay in bed, hating to breathe, all that kept looping in my mind for weeks was the act of a police officer putting my report into the trashcan and picking up the phone. I thought it was strange that he kept telling me I should think about what I was doing before I made a decision.

I don't know how I made it through those weeks of life. My first conscious thought was never again would I allow that to happen. I realized my instincts were warning me that despite what others thought, my gut knew he was too connected to the authorities.

I deserve to be loved

Herein you can see a shift in my thinking that would change my life and focus. I did a lot of "getting real with myself" while staring into my past, present and future possibilities. I deserve a life better than my current circumstances. It wasn't my fault I had no family to protect me. It would be my fault if I didn't defend myself and my daughter.

I decided to listen to the mantra of nature with the birds singing a song of work and play. The rain was creating a storm that resounded in my heart. On my back, begging heaven to stop the pain, I finally accepted that this was where my body was at that time.

It hurt, but I would overcome. It was scary, but I would find a way to prosperity. Most importantly, it was not going to happen again. With that thought I rested my case. It didn't occur again when he came back; I was ready.

Victory Day

Oh, this day sealed is in my memory. I spent three months diligently building my confidence and a plan.

The door to my house was unlocked because I was about to leave. He walked in. I was at the top of the stairs, with only a long dress like a sheath for protection. My daughter was in her room, I gave the verbal signal for her to lock up her bedroom.

I had planned this moment to be whatever it needed to be to get the job done. I looked outside. It was a cold October day with the sun shining bright. The sun beamed like lasers through the trees. One single thought resonated in my mind "It's either him or me, and it's not going to be me today." In that moment I defined my life going forward, it was the decision that changed my stars forever.

It was so easy to breathe. I felt a rising of determination inside. I let it come; it wasn't the emotion of hate, anger, or fear. Instead, absolute conviction resolve of purpose, and all of my attention went to being the huntress. The protectress invoked. I didn't feel violent and I wasn't trembling. I knew what my body could stand. My mind was razor-sharp. I wanted this challenge to be born into me.

He called out, "Bitch, don't look at me like that."

I reached inside to my inner power and let it rise to my eyes. I wasn't going to hide. Then I smiled. He put up his fist, telling me I was going to get a beating for showing disrespect. I walked towards him in my dress, looking him dead soul center in the eyes and staring right at his inner demon, his dysfunctional personality, and his depraved drugged mind.

A feeling of strength poured into me like warm water. It was almost sexy in its feminine sovereignty. I was sure I would endure. I responded, "No matter what you do today, I will use everything to put you six feet under hell." I stood right in front of him on the fourth step right within the fist range. I had already calculated several different moves, and the counter moves to keep my ribs safe. I had a camera at the ready with a state trooper officer number from another state I had picked out to call, someone who looked like he ate drug dealers for lunch.

I felt my eyes change, and my scent became like an animal, the only warning he would ever get. I would marvel at that experience later. Then the magic happened; his eyes, those which had plagued me for so many years, suddenly shifted to fear. I saw it as a flash of insight across his face; his time was over. He was done tormenting me by my decree — not his, not the universe, nor society — my choice for my life.

To my shock, he looked terrified, gazed behind me then ran out the door. All that remained was only squealing tires, dust in the driveway and one gone psychopath from my life. My daughter and I danced, laughing in each other's arms on our momentous occasion. It was a race no one would ever see — a victory up a mountain of unscalable proportions. It was a beginning and an end.

He stayed gone. I found out last April that he died.

What is resilience?

To me, it's the song of knowledge in us that we are destined to become the most excellent version of self beyond our conscious limitations. Complimentary compatible and genius. An ultimate design of power, manifested through learning. Resilience is taking back our fierceness with force at times and laughing in relief at others.

You are meant to have a paradise life of epic experience. This truth, when the mind accepts it, forms a barrier to any obstacle. Giving unlimited strength at the time you need it the most — the moment when you might otherwise give in to the lie of defeat. We are made to challenge that which contests our right to victory.

Whether it's resisting the temptation to fill up our frenzied emotions with food, drink, distraction, or toxic choices, we have all we need to overcome. Fearing a fist, insult, or loss, regardless of what challenges your worthiness in the moment, it's in our nature to respond like a champion.

Breathe in and out; there's your channel of the integrity of form and masterful strength. Next, think I am made for epic greatness. Breathe in and out; there is the mental link of aptitude. Sit for a moment in gratitude for every cell of your body shining light, pulsing the message, "I've got you at this moment. You are not alone in this conscious place of concepts and kinetic matter." Something inherently yours is determining in every moment that you are worthy of life. A potent truth I have come to in all of my choices, those I embraced and ones I ran from screaming on the inside, it all came down to this: the purpose of resilience is to ensure that we never forget our self-worth. Our inherent beauty, in all forms of loving expression, is our compass.

Everyone has a story of struggle, challenge, and a cross-roads of contemplation. I assure you that on the other side of your sorrow is a profound victory and solace from all that derives from pain. One of the most significant ways you can change the momentum of life is to turn the absence of good into a mission to make the world better.

I have a magnum opus of desire to make the world a safer place for orphans and children. My experiences have shaped my life, and I won't apologize for being who I am. The same courage and determination that walked down a flight of stairs can walk up to receive a universal reward of blessings and abundance.I am to become a Paradise Maker life.

I have a new vision to build a network of role models that provide a service for family security. A platform to encourage and sustain the strong masculine example of legacy greatness. Handsome, strong, intelligent, and spiritually aligned men walk the earth, making a difference every day. I'm determined to support them and give them more ways to serve. One day in the future, stalkers won't exist, orphans mistreated will be of the past. Men and women will live in the genius design of complementary compatibility, which creates a fulfilling family legacy. I will be part of the solution and drive to give my children that future.

I encourage you to find your mission of might that makes all of your moments not in vain! Now live the strength of your bones with no excuses; your body deserves the experience of living in victory. Give yourself the triumph of love in life!

About the Author

Alexsa Covelli rose from the challenge of being orphaned at birth and fostered in a home that believed being ambidextrous with a high IQ was akin to evil. She channeled her quest for a better life into art and design, initially building a career in interior design with prominent professionals, which included her discreet specialized approach of relationship crisis management to doctors and high-level executives with burnout.

After becoming a widow she needed a shift of focus. Being a lifelong learner, she took a sabbatical to travel and experience a new level of inspiration. She added pre- and post-natal coaching, fitness coaching and Breatheology coaching to her skill sets. She now writes full time, stays fit with her TYTAX, and enjoys raising three children.

Her mission is to use her creative drive to be a catalyst for new social possibilities supporting positive role models in the modern evolution of our time. As an advocate for family security her dream is to build a sanctuary of excellence for the next generation of Morphans. Orphans who morph into excellence from the challenge of coming into the world alone.

Tips to cultivate calm confidence

Confidence is a quality we can all develop in small steps and practices that help us to get calm and centered are well worth exploring. When we can manage our own physiology, it gives us more belief in ourselves and it also helps us to manage anxiety, worry and panic.

Start by recalling a time when you felt really resilient, confident and in charge of your own emotions. What gave you this sense of confidence? What helped you to manage your emotions? How did embodying resilience help you feel? What led to this situation?

See if you can find nuggets of information that help you identify qualities you may have forgotten you possess. This will help to boost your confidence and self-belief without too much effort!

Scenario rehearsal

Some people find scenario rehearsal useful to help them feel more confidently about a situation.

If you can't help but think the worst, get calm with deep breathing or a short meditation focused on your breath and then allow yourself to imagine the worst possible scenario. Remember as you do this, that you are safe and make sure you keep breathing slowly whilst you let your mind conjure up images.

Bring to mind everything that could go wrong, then imagine yourself handling every tough moment with grace. In other words, imagine how the best version of you would confidently work through the problem without failing.

Based on this, make a list of at least three ways you could handle negative situations in future, to bring about a positive outcome whilst maintaining your cool.

Get grounded

Sometimes, the simple act of getting out of your own head by grounding your energy, can be enough to give you a sense of calm confidence.

The easiest way to do this is to drop your attention down to your feet, noticing the surface underneath them and the feel of socks and shoes if you're wearing them. Wriggle your toes to help you sense into your feet. Notice that whilst you do this, your head tends to get quieter. It can also be helpful to picture a wide beam of light or a wide tree trunk going down into the earth underneath your feet. Imagine that with each inhalation, you are drawing nourishment and strength into your body from the earth.

Use your breath

Our lungs are our interchange between the outer and inner worlds. They help us to process toxins, energize our system and keep us healthy. There is a reason that the practice of Pranayama, or yoga breathing, has survived for centuries, and that is because it offers an intentional way to invigorate and recharge you.

When you practice slow breathing for a few moments daily, you regain a sense of calm control over yourself. Intentional breaths are much fuller than our default breathing pattern and when you consciously breathe for a few moments, you will feel calmer, more grounded and much more present.

Try the practice of Square Breathing for a few minutes when you wake up, ensuring you are sitting upright to give your lungs more space to expand.

Place your hands on your belly to help you breathe in more fully and then repeat four simple breath sections through your nose, to a count of four as below. When you pause, stay as relaxed in your shoulders and upper chest as you can and repeat as many times as you like. Use this breath whenever you want to feel calmer and more confident.

1. Inhale 2 3 4
2. Hold 2 3 4
3. Exhale 2 3 4
4. Hold 2 3 4

This is a great technique to use when you feel nervous or fearful — keep breathing through the nerves and it will change your mental state.

Resilience Trait # 7
Positive Self-talk

Positive self-talk is an effective and essential tool when it comes to becoming more resilient, because it helps you to overcome the influence of your negative inner voice and your inbuilt negativity bias.

Generally speaking, we are not brought up to see ourselves as the incredible individuals we are, because growing up, we are taught to focus more on the areas where we are lacking. As children, most of us were told to 'knuckle down', 'pull up our bootstraps' and work harder. As adults, this means many of us subconsciously believe we are not good enough, a belief which is reinforced by our inner negative voice telling us stories.

You may be an extremely positive person, but your brain will still constantly look out for potential threats to your survival, registering negatives much more quickly than positives. This makes you predisposed to feel the pain of loss far more acutely than you ever experience the joy of having the same thing. Your brain has evolved to react and learn quickly from negative experiences, whereas happy ones barely register, so you have to work harder to overcome your negative beliefs.

World leading psychiatrist and neuroscientist Dr. Daniel Amen created a wonderful approach to help his patients retrain their brain to notice more positives than negatives. Recognizing that his patients unknowingly let their Automatic Negative Thoughts (ANTs) run rampant in their head, he created ANT therapy to help them eradicate their ANTs with positivity spray.

To stop the nasty little gremlin in our head from littering our brain with ANTs and robbing us of our confidence, we have to learn to disempower our thoughts. They have only as much power as we give them so we need to remember this and learn to catch them before they deplete us of our joy.

Reframing and recognizing that the negative thoughts are assumptions and stories is a powerful way to start disentangling from them.

The wiser part of you that knows how capable you are will support you as you start to identify and question each thought. As you do this, remember that you are like every other human. We all run stories in our heads without realizing it and this doesn't make us failures or weak people. It is how we are wired to make sense of the world.

The types of stories you are likely to have running habitually in your head are likely to include things like:

"I'll never be good enough for my partner."

"I'm such a mess. I'll never be good at anything."

"I'm always late."

"I'm lazy and unmotivated and there's no point starting anything."

None of these stories is helpful or encouraging and when a story reinforces negative feelings about yourself that are not necessarily true, they deplete your life force energy and demotivate you. These kind of thoughts also rewrite reality because they automatically add assumptions to your experiences. Without realizing it, you may judge others based on your own erroneous thoughts, fall into rumination because you feel inferior, or create non-existent scenarios in your head.

No matter what your inner voice says, you have not failed, you are enough and you do have what it takes to build your resilience and thrive, rather than just survive. When you learn to identify, challenge and disprove your negative thoughts, you will be able to replace the voice in your head with positive, supportive and compassionate thoughts instead.

The story presented in this chapter by Joana Soares provides wonderful insights on how to replace the negative voice in the head, along with the doubtful and pessimistic thoughts with positive self-talk and an empowering mindset. Despite being the youngest author in this book, Joana possesses a level-headed wisdom that will inspire you to look at your life with fresh eyes and stay positive on your life journey.

Seeing My Future
by Joana Soares

I've heard the call, "It's time to change".

In my bed at night, I asked myself, "If everything was possible, if you changed your current place of work, where would you go?" And then I got my answer in a magazine, a renowned veterinary hospital in my hometown, Porto, Portugal. I managed the how and made the change. Yet here I am on a bright and sunny day, feeling miserable, broken, full of despair, and filled with doubt about my work and my value as a veterinarian. A feeling that hurt so deeply that I was experiencing heart palpitations and started questioning if, what at another time has been my dream career, being able to save animals and to be with animals everyday, should even be my profession.

I've lost my previous home in the south of Portugal, Algarve, where I've lived for three years and come back to my parents' house. My boyfriend, Luís, had lost his job because of me. I was not feeling welcomed or supported at work, I had no friends there, and I was feeling like a machine, seeing animal after animal like I was in an assembly line, so quickly that I haven't even learned their names. That was killing me inside. I knew I had to do something.

I remember asking for the universe's help. I heard, "Now you know more, Joana". Then I started to see my personal sign, which is the color blue turquoise in some of my patients' collars, which told me, "You are on the right path". I also saw some dogs who were very similar to and had the same name as my beloved first dog, Lucky. She was the reason why I chose veterinary school in the first place.

I started to do some guided meditations, to listen to some inspiring audios and videos, and to search for inspiring quotes. I repeated a five minute audio program of affirmations right before work, which was very helpful with my anxiety. I also made an effort to focus on all the positive things in my life. For example, I was able to be with my grandmother everyday and enjoy her food, I had my family with me again, I had a roof over my head and a comfortable bed, an income, a loving partner, etc. I started to exercise with a personal trainer and that has improved my energy and health.

During that shifting moment I remember I received a message from my previous receptionist telling me that my clients from my previous job were asking for me and telling her how loved I was by them and their pets, and that all my coworkers and friends missed me. That message gave me a lot of strength. To support my self-worth and the knowledge I was doing my best, working with pets and their families, I created a list of my "success" cases, including every animal I've saved. That gave me a lot of motivation and courage to face my current situation.

Then magic started to happen. I was offered a ticket to go to a congress in Lisbon, and guess who was there? My previous boss and one of my best friends and colleagues from the south. I discovered there was a spot available in that hospital, my spot. Something inside of me was telling me, you have to go back. And so I did. All of my family members supported me, and my beloved Luís turned his life upside down for me again, for that I am forever grateful.

Coming back was amazing; all my friends were there, my clients, my support system, my work family, and I loved Algarve's climate and landscapes so much. Luís found a better job that he likes and we were having a splendid spring and summer.

In September 2018 came one of my biggest challenges in life, I had my first panic attack after a discussion with some colleagues because I was trying to protect an animal. That part was really tough for me. I contacted my beloved psychologist, and she also said "Joana, you know more now".

How could I have almost burned myself out? How could I forget myself again? Why can't I defend my clients, the animals, and what I believe in without being aggressive and misunderstood? I started to meditate again, everyday, taking care of myself. I took some vacation time afterwards and I was feeling better. But sometimes a little voice was whispering: "You are supposed to do more, outside of the hospital, besides being a veterinary doctor doing consultations. You're made to help in another dimension, on a bigger stage. You have to do more, to help more".

I ignored that voice as I didn't know how to do it, where to start... I continued to distract myself with my "everyday life", stressing out with little problems, stressful shifts, almost forcing Luís to marry me because I felt we were supposed to do that since we are near thirty, and a lot of other negative things. Sometimes when the little voice whispered, "maybe you could start by doing some YouTube videos, by teaching what you know about animals" quickly I answered "when I have time", "maybe when I have a baby and I'll be at home".

But I guess the Universe knows what it is doing. In April 2019 I was working on a night-shift at the hospital and boom! Suddenly I was blind in my left eye. I had discovered in 2011 that I have a rare congenital problem in my left eye, but back then I was seeing 10/10 so I could live perfectly well with that condition. My doctor had prepared me by telling me that if one day I stopped seeing I had to go immediately to the emergency room because it could be a displaced retina. And so it was.

Because I know how to react in emergency situations (actually it is one of my gifts) I sat down and started to breathe deeply, again and again. When I felt calmer, I asked for help and began to draw up a plan. We were calling all hospitals to know which ones took ophthalmology emergencies, but none did.

So I left the veterinary hospital with Luís and we went to the biggest hospital in Algarve, but still no one knew what to do. I kept on breathing and as soon as I could, I took the next train to Porto to see my doctor. I had a retina displacement, but not "the normal kind". This problem happens because there is liquid inside of the layers of the retina, which is much more complicated to solve.

Because I got better from one day to another (with less liquid) I escaped surgery, and I was at home in bed for two to three weeks. During that period I had a lot of time to think. *What am I not seeing? Is it the way I'm leading my relationship with Luis? My deep mission in life? I have to love myself more? I'm not seeing my superpowers?*

The doctor said I was better so I came back to the south. During that week, my mother and grandmother were with me. I was at home, I rested and some friends came to visit me but I was feeling sad, nervous and anxious. I started to think about work problems again, I didn't know how to come back and deal with some situations that were happening. I even had two job proposals, which confused me.

Another doctor's appointment and my eye relapsed. And you know what? I was invited to go to an event in Alicante, Spain called ETTG (The European Transformational Teachers Gathering). There I would meet my lovely mentor Dr. Andrea Pennington[1], with whom I previously had the opportunity to write a book called *Time to Rise*. I also met Charlotte Banff,[2] an animal healer and communicator, the founder of the "Animal Healer Academy", with whom I had the opportunity to start my learning on her foundation course. I met a lot of other beautiful colleagues from our magical tribe.

I wasn't sure I should travel to Spain with this eye problem. But surprisingly my doctor said, "yes, you can go", in fact three doctors did. And now, I'm so glad and grateful I had the courage to make that trip. In Spain I had some of the best days of my life. I opened my heart while going through suffering, longing, and reflection[3]. I learnt beautiful things, I heard amazing stories, had a lot of insights, and meet wonderful people. I felt so loved, so protected, so inspired. I came out with a lot of awareness. I am where I am supposed to be, everything happens for a reason.

During that magical event I meet a special soul brother named Javier[4] who offered me two crystals; one for protection and another one which I meditate with and had an unlocking moment. I also meet a musician named Paul Luftnegger,[5] whose music will change the world because it is profound, healing and beautiful. I left Spain with my cup running over, my heart full of love, and feeling prepared for what would come next.

I had to go to surgery. The day of the operation I felt so peaceful, so protected, and everything went well. After surgery I had to be in a very uncomfortable position with my head down for two weeks, using a special chair. This made it very difficult to sleep. Music helped a lot, as did meditation and the nursing care of my grandmother. I listened to a lot of inspirational podcasts and heard a lot of YouTube videos. My creativity was on fire; I even managed to feel little moments of bliss and happiness while listening to music, holding hands with my grandmother, and writing down my ideas to help animals and people. I planned to create videos, workshops, and to start spreading my knowledge with a higher purpose and mission.

In this tough period of my life, I discovered how resilient I am, and how you can be too:

1. Be truthful to yourself, get to know you
2. Do affirmations, meditate, listen to music
3. Get help, focus on a good outcome
4. FORGIVE
5. Believe it's possible, become ready
6. Go back to nature, be with your animals and loved ones
7. Be passionate about what you love, be grateful
8. Be strong, feel love, be love
9. Take action, be light, be your own healer
10. Never give up!

Although after the first surgery the eye problem was unsolved (I still had some liquid, the retina was detached, and I was seeing very badly) the doctor said I could go back to my normal life. Only time would return my eye to normal. And so I returned to my life. I was so happy to see my boyfriend and my four pawed family members again (my cat named Mia and my dog, Sasha). I was enjoying nature, seeing trees (and new colors) I never paid attention to before. Sometimes it felt like an "after-trauma" reaction, reliving some memories about the last time I was home, but I was able to control my mind and be at a state of peace and gratitude again. I was planning to go back to work as a new Joana, focussing on what matters, the wellbeing of my patients, the reason I do what I do (a deep will to help and save animals) and I was planning to act on my own ideas for a business. I've worked with David Dorotea[6], my Portuguese coach and we've found a big goal to pursue.

One late afternoon, I started to see "flies" with my left eye. Deep inside I knew something was going wrong, so I called my doctor and was advised to go to the emergency room, again. My retina had ruptured from the top. Oh no!

There I reached my rock bottom. A place of sadness, despair, and grief. A special friend told me to look inside my eyes, to search for divine help. Crying on the ground looking in the mirror I prayed for help, and nothing. *Let's face reality; I have to go to Porto again,* seven hours by train. Because it was not the first time, I knew what to do to make myself (and my family) calm. During the trip I felt a strong will to write a poem, and so I did. The message of strength, peace, and faith was there. It felt like a message from God.

The next day I was going to my second surgery. All that positioning again. At least I have my music, my audios, my friends praying for me and sending me healing vibes and love, and my family supporting me. The day before surgery, another special friend named Gitte[7] told me about my third eye and guided me to look beyond. This time, on the night of the surgery, in a meditative state, I received a message from the angels and from my grandparents who had passed away. I finally saw my "woo-woo superpowers".

The recovery period after my second surgery was very different, much more of an inner work, a battle with myself. How did I do it? I was blessed and helped in a lot of different ways. I got in contact with my higher-self and learned to love myself deeply, from inside-out[8]. I opened my heart. I began to repeat "I am enough" everyday[9].

I held on to my resilience and previous lessons. I've followed my intuition everyday. I've listened to what I felt was right at the moment (a lot of Paul's music) and I learned about unconditional love[10]. I've forgiven all the people that hurt me with a special healing help[11]. I've practised Louise Hay's[12] affirmations and saw her movie. I've followed her advice to "Rise like a Phoenix". I've heard my mentors and friends (thank God for you, Andrea[1]). I've practised gratitude and acceptance.

I was ready to receive love, light and a cure from above. I believed. I've moved forward despite my fears, and I've released them. I took my power back, since I began to believe that **I am my own healer**. Finally, I saw what it is really being a LovePair of God, living a human experience.

On June 11th I reached the point of no return; I'm not the same Joana anymore, I'm a medium, I am a rider of the blessed possessions and the animal kingdom, and my mission is to help animals and people around the world honoring and serving our planet earth with divine help. I also received purple orchids that day to celebrate. The next day the doctor said my eye was substantially better.

I'm healed now and I see clearly. I see a world of possibilities. I see love, joy, truth, peace, light, magic, hope, beauty, goodness, tenderness, dreams, health, prosperity, and abundance. I see the sky, the sea, nature, animals, our planet earth needing help and unconditional love. I see all the Lightworkers coming together.

Would you like to come with us?

With love,
Joana

This is a list of the beautiful souls who have supported me on this healing journey. I am deeply grateful for their presence in my life.

[1] Andrea Pennington
[2] Charlotte Banf
[3] Anja Holmbäck
[4] Javier Martinez
[5] Paul Luftnegger
[6] David Dorotea
[7] Gitte Winter Graugaard
[8] Kevin Froystad
[9] Marisa Peer
[10] Sólveig Þórarinddóttir
[11] Elspeth Kerr
[12] Louise Hay

About the Author

Whether people see it or not, the reality is a lot of animals around the world are deeply suffering because they are being mistreated, or simply misunderstood. Veterinarian Joana Soares is on a mission to help change that reality.

Joana is a passionate, dedicated, intuitive doctor of animals, first inspired by her own dog, Lucky, and her special interest is in helping pets and their owners to form a deeply connected bond. With a strong connection they can intuitively communicate or "tune in together" to support each other on their mutual healing journey.

She accepted this pioneering calling when she started noticing a strong correlation between the health of pets, their owners and their families during her clinical observations. This became the foundational idea behind Joana's innovative concept of the LovePair, which focuses on the love, compassion and communication between pets and owners as an important contributor to their respective wellbeing.

To connect with Dr. Joana Soares write to joanarsoares12@gmail.com or join her facebook group www.facebook.com/groups/2065145523728670/

Tips to Knock Out Negative Self-Talk and Bring Out Your Inner Cheerleader

The negative voice in our head is a nasty little gremlin that robs us of our confidence, but luckily, we also have an inner cheerleader.

As you discovered in the introduction to this chapter, the most effective way to take our power back from our inner gremlin is to identify, challenge and disprove our negative thoughts. You can then replace them with positive, supportive, compassionate thoughts so that you shift the balance in favor of your inner cheerleader.

This is a practice that gets easier and more habitual over time and is well worth persisting with. Use your breath to breathe through any discomfort or challenging emotions.

I. Become aware of the mental script in the background of your life.

Which phrases do you hear often?

Do you engage in any self name calling, like "dummy or idiot?"

How about the tone of the voice in your head? Is the voice nasty and mean?

Are the words familiar to you from your childhood?

II. Question and challenge the voices

Ask yourself, "Is it true?" And be honest with yourself!

If you feel it is true, ask yourself how you know this to be true.

III. Disprove the inner commentary

Expose the lies by finding evidence to the contrary. If this is challenging, ask yourself what evidence there is to prove it is true - because there won't be any.

For example, if you hear an inner voice saying, "I always mess up!"

Look for evidence in your life where you did not mess up. You may have messed up sometimes, but think of all the times when you didn't, that your inner voice has conveniently chosen to ignore.

IV. Replace the lies with truth.

Remind yourself that you are competent, smart, helpful and worthy of success.

Remind yourself of all your wins and successes. Gather physical evidence if this helps, such as thank you notes, testimonials, messages of support and gratitude.

Create a personal success mantra, a positive affirmation of truth about you. It can be useful to base this around quotes and phrases that inspire you and elevate your mood.

V. Take positive action to affirm your power.

Go out and prove your case. Use your talents and abilities in a new, different or challenging way.

Extra Tips:

To help you identify your thoughts, it can be helpful to carry a journal or notebook with you, so that you can make a note of any negative thoughts you notice during the day. Creating a regular journaling practice is also an extremely good way to make friends with your own mind and allow it to offload any concerns. There is no right or wrong way to do this, just make sure sure that you don't get dragged into rumination or get caught in the trap of chastising yourself.

Another useful practice is to short-circuit negative thoughts as soon as you notice them arising. Choosing a phrase as simple as "Stop" is an effective way to get better at noticing these insidious thoughts.

Finally, do something small every day to honor yourself. This could be adopting a new positive daily habit, making sure you smile at a stranger every day, having a more mindful shower or cooking yourself healthy food.

Resilience Trait # 8
Connection to Positive
People

It can be tempting to withdraw from the world when we are stressed, but prolonged isolation can keep us stuck in negativity. The most resilient people make sure that they find like-minded, positive people for social support, because this helps them to maintain a positive outlook and enjoy life.

When you cannot see the wood for the trees, you need a helping hand to shift your focus back onto the steps you can take — even if they are small ones. Any action is better than no action if you want to move forwards, so leaning on your positive friends for ideas will help boost your resilience.

Positive people lift you up and reinforce your belief in the power of hope and possibility and when you face challenges, these are qualities you want to reminded of. Whilst many people, including me, like to be alone when they're stressed, over time this reduces the likelihood of you bouncing back. Resilient people lean on and into positive relationships and this helps you to stay healthier and cope better with stressful situations.

When you surround yourself with positive people, they have the emotional intelligence to give you space when you need it, as well as listen and gently challenge you when it will serve you better. Because positive people choose to live in a more empowered way, they are unlikely to try and solve your problems for you, minimize them or add fuel to any dramas you experience. Positive people respect other people and they honor your innate intelligence rather than try to offer you advice.

When you feel stuck and lost for any reason, you need support from people who can help you shift your state and change your perspective. There is nothing worse than getting so caught up in your own emotions and problems that you feel powerless to make changes. Studies show that a sense of belonging is extremely important for emotional health and well-being; for example, those who have social support but don't feel they truly belong, are much more likely to suffer from depression. (Cohen, S. Social Relationships and Health. American Psychologist. 2004)

You have probably heard the phrase 'you are the average of the five people you spend most time with', attributed to motivational speaker Jim Rohn. It references the fact that humans are wired to emulate behaviors in social groups to help them integrate, so we unknowingly adapt to fit in with others around us. When we realize that the people we spend most time with influence us, we can shift our focus to spending more time with those we most strongly resonate with.

Make a conscious effort to find the people who love and accept you for who you are, share your values, elevate you, give you a sense of accountability and positively influence the choices you make.

If you struggle to find those people in the real world, see if you can find them online. If this fails, shift your perspective to focus on what you can control and influence — make the decision to be the positive person in the room, smile and shine your light so brightly that those seeking positive people will find you.

Our first story illustrating the importance of forging positive connections so that we can build resilience, is from an inspirational mentor who went from having it all to his entire life crumbling. This captivating story shares how Rob Goddard almost dramatically let everything go, after falling into deep depression and failing to turn his life around. With help from a man he calls his "angel", the author was given the opportunity to view his life from a different perspective so that he could start visualizing and creating a more positive and fulfilling future.

In our second story, we discover how deeply a sense of disconnection in childhood underpins how we subsequently operate as adults. This story is from a kind-hearted author, Mona Winbrant, who did everything she could as a child to stay quiet, fit in and please others. Her desire to avoid passing on her childhood patterns to her own children eventually led to her ignoring her own needs so much, she experienced burnout. In this story, she shares her subsequent journey to reconnecting to her deepest self and to others and the discoveries and learnings she made along the way.

The connection you have to 'Mother Nature' can also provide resilience boosting support. While she is not a person, per se, being in nature can provide much needed insight, clarity and loving support. In fact this first story about such a connection is from a sensitive and creative woman who quite literally lost sight of her most fundamental connections and practices. As a result or trying to be all things to all people, Lene Kirk's life slowly shifted from being mindful and manageable to being extremely stressful. This story shares how accessing resilience in small steps took the her from being unable to move or see much, to being vibrantly alive and full of joy. It illustrates how powerful the connection between our body, mind and heart are and how positively we can impact our entire lives by honoring that connection, along with our connection to nature.

From Suicide to Success
by Robert Goddard

In 2010, I was on the 125th floor of the world's tallest building, the Burj Khalifa tower in Dubai, preparing for my death. For months I had searched the internet looking for painless ways to kill myself. I decided on jumping from a great height. I calculated that it would only take me 13 seconds to fall nearly 3,000 feet. Then it would all be over. It could be even sooner than that as I had read that I was likely to have a heart attack on the way down. No more pain, nor struggling, just nothing.

Just two years earlier, I was in the top 1% of earners in the UK. I was 45 years old and in the prime of my life. I had a lovely home, wife and twin boys, and I was highly successful in business. I felt invincible in life, like I was made of granite rock.

However, in a 3-month period in the summer of 2008, my life crumbled. I lost my marriage, my children and my job. I went into an emotional tailspin. I fell out of the sky like an eagle that had been shot by an unknown sniper from the ground. I had never been out of work in my life and as a result I felt like a complete failure in life because I couldn't provide for my family. The centre of my world had been my career and the materialism that surrounded it. I was in a complete state of shock and bewilderment.

Extreme anxiety set in which led me to stop sleeping or eating at all, for days. My mind was in perpetual turmoil trying to process what had happened and how I could sort the whole mess out. I would stare at the TV screen for long periods and not remember what I had just watched. The only thing that filled my waking and non-waking hours was the constant, torturous churn of my disastrous situation.

The day I lost my job I went to see my doctor to get some medication to help me get through this shock. In her office, I broke down. In floods of tears and broken sentences I managed to get out that I had come to the end of my life and didn't know where to turn. She was empathetic and promised that a counselling service would contact me. Then she handed me a bewildering and colourful array of pills. I thought to myself, "Once the drugs take effect, I'll be back to my normal self within a couple of weeks and then I can start to rebuild my life again."

I didn't know that what lay ahead of me was a 5-year battle with depression and me repeatedly feeling that suicide was the only way out. Fortunately, I did meet an "angel" and I'd like to introduce you to him later.

My situational depression was like a black menacing cloud. It came and went as it wanted for many years, affecting my emotions and my mind. I didn't talk to anyone about it, I was too ashamed of feeling the way I did. So, I just put on a brave face, a mask, to the outside world. Contrary to what you may think, it's not suicide that kills, it's the loneliness and isolation. Here's the dichotomy, in a highly connected modern world, we can isolate ourselves so easily. Most depressed people don't want to be a burden on others.

Instead, they just suffer in silence and some, sadly, in desperation take their life.

Did you know that 2,200 people a day commit suicide every year on this planet? That's up 40% over the past two decades! Of those, 75% are men. Many men are far worse at expressing their feelings than women. We often lock things away, don't speak up and sometimes the dam breaks. We have a global crisis on our hands. Suicide is the biggest killer of people aged under 45 in the UK. I would have been one of those statistics had events not gone a different route.

by 2010 my life hadn't bounced back, I was still being prescribed drugs by the doctor, but by then I had started to self-medicate with alcohol. Vodka was a quick way of making my mind go fuzzy for a few hours so that I could forget my depression, albeit temporarily. Eventually I stopped taking the prescribed drugs and started stockpiling them instead. In the end I had over 700 pills tucked away in my wardrobe, a secret stash. I thought that if I couldn't control what happened in my life anymore, at least I could determine when and how my life ended. At least I had that control remaining in my life.

Because of regular anxiety attacks, I had numerous restless nights, tossing and turning like a ship caught at sea in an unforgiving storm. I started waking up later, I would keep my dressing gown on throughout the day. I didn't eat properly, didn't shave, and rarely washed. I must have stunk! I had become a functioning alcoholic.

Self-employment was forced upon me, I had no choice. I did manage to slowly build a small business, but it was very tough. I remember travelling to sales pitch meetings with music blaring out of the car's speakers, crying my eyes out en-route, only to discreetly park around the corner from the offices, wipe my eyes and my nose, then put on a mask. I also had a stash of mints in the car to mask the smell of vodka, which I popped before entering the building. I became an "actor" for a couple of hours.

But life just bumped along the bottom, I was just surviving and definitely not thriving. Then, out of the blue my main client terminated our contract and my life again spun immediately out of control. Once again I looked at the dark abyss opening up in front of me.

A fresh start

So, in March 2010, I decided to run away to the bright and alluring lights of Dubai to become a Financial Adviser, with the invitation to a job that would provide untold riches for me, or so they promised. In reality, it was a commission only job, working in a part of the world I have never been to and in a culture which I had never encountered previously. It was an opportunity to prove to myself once again that I could bounce back. I had worked in Financial Services for three decades, I believed I could really do it, again.

Initially, I was so full of energy, enthusiasm and renewed hope when I went to see my new Regional Director, at the glitzy Dubai Marina. He was half my age but had been in the country for 4 years and was the top salesman in the company, he had a boat in the Marina and a Porsche 911. At last, a blank canvas, a fresh start where nobody knew me. It may have been commission only and living in one of the most expensive cities in the world, but I was up for the challenge.

I started my new job with no data, no client base, no website, no marketing budget, just me and a bunch of business cards and a winning smile! I figured that my target market included expatriates, high net worth individuals who paid no tax and were dripping with surplus cash. So, I decided to go where they tend to hang out, meet them, chat and make myself visible. Places like the Yacht Marina, the Irish pub Fibber's McGee, The Polo Club and the prestigious car dealerships like Ferrari, Lamborghini, Porsche, even the Harley Davidson dealership. I also used LinkedIn, creating a stream of articles on "hot topics" of interest to some of the worlds' richest people, positioning myself as a "thought leader" in all matters financial. Leads started to flood in, new clients were signing up and at last I was making some serious money again.

However, I had completely underestimated trying to fit in with an immensely fast-moving society and, what seemed to me at least, was a superficial and uncaring environment. A micro climate where people rarely had the time or inclination to build real friendships. At the same time, I had also cut myself off from my family and my close friends, working in a country 3,500 miles away.

The blazing summer sun was like an inferno and coupled with the stifling humidity of Dubai, it was like working in my own hell. I felt like a prisoner condemned to a life of hard labour, paying for my heinous crimes. The money wasn't bringing happiness at all, I was gradually feeling alone in the metropolis. Isolated from family and close friends. It was a prison of my own making, albeit a golden one.

I gradually sunk into what felt like quicksand. The more I struggled against it, the more I got sucked into it. So, I kept what I called a "death diary." It was me journaling about my innermost thoughts, fears and anxieties. It helped to write things down, but the main aim was to leave something behind for my children, so that they would know why their Dad had killed himself. I didn't want them to blame themselves or think they could have done something to change the situation.

After months of battling on my own, I eventually gave up the fight. I was emotionally exhausted and battle weary, so I decided to go to the daunting and imposing tower of the Burj Khalifa, to find my way outside to jump. Thirteen seconds away from ending the pain and private hell that had become my life.

I woke up one morning and decided that today would be the day this torment would end. I showered and shaved like any normal day. I then phoned a work colleague and said that I wanted to visit the Burj Khalifa and take some pictures from the top of the tower, because despite working in Dubai, I never had time to do the tourist thing. I never disclosed to him my plan because I didn't want him to talk me out of it.

I met him at the front entrance, bought the tickets and joined the snaking queue of sightseers making their way to the lifts. As we travelled the 90 seconds to the top I recall having this macabre thought that it would only take me 13 seconds to come back down. I was calm, not stressing about what I was about to do. It was a surreal frame of mind to be in, having made the decision to end my pain. I felt empowered somehow to be taking control of my life.

We got to the 125th floor and wandered around the viewing platform with a multitude of tourists. I asked my friend to take some pictures of me looking out at the Dubai scenery and then excused myself to the bathroom. I told him I wouldn't be long. Instead, I went around the tower looking for a way to the outside of the building. The viewing platforms are floor to ceiling thick glass, so I had to find an exit that workers use to gain access to the outside of the tower.

I quickly found a fire exit and tentatively tried the handle. It was locked! Who on earth locks a fire exit door? This one was and so my attempt at suicide that day had been thwarted. I went back to my apartment, dejected, miserable and angry with myself. The stock pile of 700+ tablets looked more appealing.

A call for help

I'm not sure why, but I decided to call a friend of mine back in the UK. Alex and I had met at a business networking event just at the time I had first gone self-employed. There was an immediate connection between us and over a couple of years we became good friends. He was and still is a

Business Coach and crucially, he was the only person who kept in regular contact with me after I left for Dubai. He contacted me on a regular basis to see how things were going. I looked forward to our chats. Although, I didn't really share the full picture, I just tried to be upbeat.

But, following my thwarted suicide attempt earlier that day, I offered to fly him out to Dubai for a few days, so that we could speak in person and at length. To my surprise he jumped on a plane and we sat poolside at my apartment for hours on end. We also laughed incessantly. It was fun sharing time together. He also told me off when he peered in my fridge and challenged me with *"I can't see anything green, only meat and alcohol!"*

Alex asked me one question that changed the direction of my life. He asked, *"What do you **really** want to do with your life, Rob?"* Immediately, I said that I didn't know. But not put off by that, he persisted with, *"but if you did know, what would it look like?"*

What a great question. I then began to describe what I saw and said that I wanted to go back to my first love of Mergers and Acquisitions. With more prodding, visualizing and planning a potentially happy future, I subsequently made the decision to return back to the UK to start again.

I went on to envisage that by 2020 I would create a business worth £5m+, move somewhere in the Southern Mediterranean and I would teach English to children from a double-decker bus, and with the woman of my dreams.

With renewed hope and a clearer vision, I managed to pitch and secure 14 investors for my new business venture. I was then able to afford to pay myself a salary for the first time in 3 years. It's not been easy building a business from nothing, but with unwavering determination, that fledgling business has now grown into a multi-million-pound company across two continents, employing 25 people.

Nevertheless, I still had to kill a few ghosts from the past, so 3 years ago I set up a sister company in Dubai. The first time round in Dubai I was a beaten man, now when I come out of the airport terminal, I have a smile back on my face in a country that so nearly became my last resting place. Initially, I was apprehensive and unsure if I could make a business work out there, having failed previously. However, I felt much stronger than before. Because the UK business had some success, I used that as my confidence platform for the new Dubai business.

Over the years I have learnt from my mistakes of the past and have surrounded myself with trusted people that I can share myself with, people who act as sounding board, both in business and on a personal level. I've also set out to employ people better than me at things. There is a freedom in having others run the business day to day. That enabled me to have precious time back and I now own 4 businesses and don't work full time in any of them!

Retirement has allowed me to do the things I want with the people that I want to work with. I've broken the walls of that golden prison and have been teaching clients to do the same for the past 10 years. I now help business owners find an exit strategy, closing one chapter in their life and starting a new one. That's been my journey and I want to share with others how liberating that is. I also invest in other people's businesses and take on a few private clients for mentoring assignments. I have the privilege of being asked to speak at a wide range of other people's events, both in the UK and in the Gulf.

The road forward

Looking back, my resilience, the strength I found to fight back and triumph over adversity, came from speaking and sharing with others. Today I know there's no point in running away. Even in the darkest hour, it's healthier to just face-up and reach out in dark times.

My relationship with money has changed too. In fact, I'm in the process of setting up a charity in order to embark on a 10-year plan to create a "living legacy." An altruistic journey to make a difference to other people's lives, through a multitude of charitable causes to those in need.

My family has expanded, I now have 6 children ranging from the ages of 25 down to 6, with two sets of twins in that beautiful tribe! Had I been successful in my suicide attempt, I would have robbed all of them of a future with their Father.

I would also never have gotten together with Kristina, the woman of my dreams, either. She is originally from Albania and we have a 2nd home there on the beach overlooking the Mediterranean Sea. We've bought a boat too and still plan to buy that Double Decker bus soon.

Retirement to me is being able to do the things I choose to do, with the people that I want to be with. I can't wait for the next 10-year vision to unfold, building a charitable foundation, with the woman of my dreams, and experiencing the joy of making a difference in life.

One final thought. If you are struggling right now and if you are in a dark, cold place, I urge you to find an "Alex".

Specifically;

- Speak up and ask for help. You will **not** be a burden on anyone. Don't let isolation win. Make that call now to a trusted person. They will be honoured that you have shared something so personal with them and that you trust them.

- Don't believe the lie in your head that the world would be a better place without you in it. Dozens of people will be devastated by you taking your own life and that will affect them for the rest of their lives. Suicide is a long-term solution to a short-term problem.

Alternatively, if life is ok for you, consider becoming an "Alex" to someone that you suspect is going through a hard time. Go for a coffee or lunch, and give them time and space to open up. Let them know you are there for them, any time, any place. Give them your listening ear, not instant fixes. You could be that one person they need to help turn things around. There is no better feeling than to know that you have been instrumental in saving someone's life, just ask my friend, Alex.

About the Author

Rob now owns 4 businesses and has transitioned from an operator to investor - a journey many entrepreneurs struggle to make. He has trained over 5,000 business leaders and brings over 35 years experience of helping business owners finish one chapter in their lives and start a new one.

His original and largest business, EvolutionCBS Ltd, is a highly successful multi-million pound advisory firm in the UK and UAE. Since 2002, Rob has been responsible for the sale of nearly 400 privately-owned UK businesses, totalling over £2 billion in transaction values.

Rob also works on more philanthropic and altruistic projects and causes, especially in the area of depression and suicide. His signature talk,"Suicide to Success," is a very personal story of his own battle with depression, leading to a suicide attempt, then fighting back to win and triumph over adversity, to lead a fulfilling life, filled with fun!

Connect with Rob online and on social media:

www.robgoddard.co.uk

www.evolutioncbs.co.uk

www.evolutioncbs.co.uk/ae

www.kingmakergroup.co.uk

email:rob.goddard@robgoddard.co.uk

LinkedIn:linkedin.com/in/robgoddard

Twitter:EvolutionCBS

Lost Connections
by Mona Winbrant

Every morning until I was seven, I made my way down the road to the home of my nanny, Anna, who was just like a grandmother to me. I remember the warm light from the kitchen window, the smell of freshly made coffee and cooked oatmeal. She was always in the kitchen wearing a dress with an apron protecting it while cooking. Her grey hair was loosely tied back. She smiled when she saw me and gave me a warm hug when I entered the kitchen. We sat down at the small respatex table on the two chairs that were placed by the kitchen window where we could look at the small sparrows on the bird's board outside. For me, this was the best time of the day. And I remember it as a safe and lovely place to be in. Here I got to be myself, surrounded by joy, playfulness and unconditional love.

Shaping my reality

Growing up in a family where it was expected that I should not be seen nor heard, I quickly developed a belief that my feelings, thoughts, and presence did not count. From the outside, everything looked perfect. The truth is that I felt forgotten, sad and alone. I often came up with imaginative stories where I saw myself fighting battles for others, becoming an inspiration, role model and protagonist. My wish for myself was to get hugs and attention, which came through as being clever and dutiful. Eventually, I established patterns of being conscientious and responsive more than using imagination and creativity. Everything was about being quiet, fitting in, playing small and doing what I thought was wanted of me.

When I was eight, we moved to a peninsula and into a beautiful new house, where I started at a small primary school with only sixty pupils. It felt safe and good, and I got a lot of positive attention as it was quite rare for newcomers to come. Most children had their mums at home. My parents were at work all day so I was coping by myself when I was not in school. But I was fine with that.

Family first

When I look back at my upbringing, I see what I call the 'good girl syndrome.' I never liked getting in trouble, which I later did in my teenage years as a different strategy to get attention. I truly hated making mistakes and made sure to get good grades. My grandpa was an organist and, God bless my parents, I do not know if they saw me as a future organist, but I learned to play the organ and I was sent to ballet classes.

Out of sight, I sat at home alone and did my homework. I got the attention I craved when the grade book passed through every summer. I continued my journey of studying and stayed home in my dark grotto. I didn't bother anyone; I never asked my parents for money and never asked anyone for any help. I dreamt of meeting Mr. Right one day, having children and giving them all the love one can get.

When I gave birth to a baby boy I felt the greatest happiness on earth. Life was perfect. This was all I had dreamt of. When baby boy number two arrived eighteen months later I became a full-time mother. I wanted to be present for them. I wanted them to experience and feel the love I felt for them. Every evening I sat with my boys reading fairy tales, enjoying the moment of familiarity and closeness. I wanted everything to be perfect for my two boys – a home in peace and harmony.

I was playing all roles from being a caring and loving mother to a father, devoted aunt, funny and crazy uncle, annoying cousins and devoted and caring grandparents. I was standing on the barricade. It was my life's mission to make my children's lives more loving, caring and joyful than I had experienced.

When the boys were 2 and 4 years old, my husband and I bought a new house and we needed more money to pay mortgages and kindergarten, so it was natural, as the champ I was, to take on the role of the family's main breadwinner. My husband used the opportunity to buy a lovely Harley Davidson, which he had always dreamt of and went out on trips. "This gives me the space and the fun I need when I am not working," he said. It made me, ultimately, feel even more tired and I noticed that I had less and less energy.

Having a bubbling sense of 'something'

Right before the summer holiday, a friend invited me to a so-called inspirational seminar. Entering the room, I saw there was a brochure on each chair saying: "Remember you are lovable, valuable and much more capable than you think you are." The female speaker came into the room, representing a strong presence and karma. I was blown away with her inspirational speech represented by her natural authority and strong authenticity. I felt she spoke directly to me and I heard her words whispering to me: "When are you going to start loving yourself? Remember, it is a choice. And it is all lined up for you!"

I immediately got this bubbly sense of zeal for richness — an eagerness for breathing, feeling my pulse, and seeking to fully live life. Even if my longing was painful, it fulfilled a purpose for me: namely, the purpose of making meaning in this life. Passions are like little treadmills of hope in the abyss. We may be going nowhere, but there is the sensation of forward motion — something to anticipate, a reason for being, a distraction from death and larger existential questions like; "What is life actually about?" and "What am I doing here?"

Running on empty

I had been successfully working in business development roles within the finance and insurance industry for the last 15 years, creating long-term value and exponential growth for the companies I worked for. On a cold winter day in January, twelve years after the birth of my second child, it was so cold that when I went out, ice crystals formed in my hair. It was as cold outside as I felt inside. On this particular morning I was on my way to the office for a meeting. During the meeting, I saw one of my colleagues standing in front of me pointing in my direction. He said, "what are you thinking? Do you have any input for us?" I wondered, "what is he talking about?" I looked at him with big eyes thinking, "I don't quite understand. Why is he standing in front of me? Why?" Suddenly I could no longer hear what he was saying, or what anyone was saying. I found myself incapable of speaking. I remember thinking, "Please, anyone, help me out here. I need to escape. I am running on empty."

The feeling of emptiness and numbness

The next day I found myself on the couch at home. The doctor had been clear "You have had enough. You're burned out." The day before I had been to my GP's office, Dr. Kaur. She was young and beautiful with classic Assyrian, Indian features. She was the child of second-generation immigrants who made sure that their children were getting an education. Typically, for the girls, they often became doctors, lawyers or other highly academic successes. Dr. Kaur appeared friendly and accommodating. "I will write you an order for three months of sick leave to begin with."

Back home, I laid down on the sofa staring at the ceiling, feeling full of shame and powerlessness, thinking I was a loser. "The good girl, who always made sure to have everything in place, being a total perfectionist, had collapsed. She had run out of fuel."

Having escaped from my husband seven years earlier to make sure we were in a safe and secure environment, I then found myself deeply depressed and with all lights burned out. I saw myself as someone who played the last act in a Greek drama. This unique play had no spectators or other fellow actors.

The body tells the truth

The feeling of solitude and isolation came quickly. Everything in the fifteen previous years of my kids' lives I had done everything to take care of them and worked hard to pay my bills. I was feeling like a caged hamster running on its wheel. In total, I had lived under pressure and high-stress levels for the previous twenty-five years, which combined with little sleep, led to struggles with concentration, and difficulties during conversations and at work. At that time I could no longer read business documents and would get very distracted quickly.

Today I am convinced that our body speaks. Our physical condition is connected to our emotions and wellbeing. I was unable to release my feelings and I am convinced it was manifested into physical challenges. Slowly, as a child, I developed conditions with high fever, eczema and asthma. Today I know, it was a scream for release and help.

The exhaustion had led to tremendous sadness and depression, where I saw little meaning in life beyond the responsibility I had for my two children. I thought at times that if only I could hang in there five more years, then the boys would be adults and able to take care of themselves. At that point, the vision for my life, was that in five more years, my boys would not need me anymore, and my mission would be completed.

Rising horizon

When the first three months of my sick leave had passed, and I found I had done nothing at all and felt worse than ever, I decided to travel to my childhood town and walk on the beach. It was a beautiful spring day, where the snow and ice had melted. At three o'clock in the afternoon it was getting dark already in Norway. These transitions often give a beautiful colour play in the sky with shifts from yellow to orange, pink and bright red, and where the cold blue heaven breaks up and makes the horizon clearer and clearer. I noticed it gave me a feeling of power and presence. I suddenly felt unbeatable.

It became clear to me; I wanted to say thank you for the invitation to join some friends traveling to Cote d'Azur on the French Riviera, to stay in the house of the late-departed painter Henri Matisse. My friends were talented painters, and I welcomed the time to paint and, sleep and relax.

Arriving at Villa Le Rève, the home of Henri Matisse, in the medieval town of Vence on the French Rivera, which was surrounded by a beautiful blooming garden and palm trees, I felt like I was stepping into a world of life, devotion and mystery. Close to the centre of Vence, you will find a sacred place which is unique in the world: The Rosary Chapel. Entirely conceived and decorated by Henri Matisse, it is an artistic marvel and considered by the painter himself as his masterpiece.

While my friends in pure euphoria started painting, I chose to concentrate on my "rehabilitation." At least until I got paintbrushes in my hand and a ready-made canvas delivered. I sat on the second floor and looked out of Matisse's balcony overlooking the Cote d'Azur, bordered by small villages with earth-coloured brick houses. I felt grief and joy. Eventually, I went into a world of flow, ecstasy, emotion, and despair, which allowed me to play with colours and techniques that I was shown along the way. "This really gives me joy and a feeling of hovering in the air like a free bird." I couldn't remember having felt anything like this.

The journey to France and the painting experience were the gateway to a universe I heard and read about. It inspired me to explore more. I signed up for a painting course, started reading books and gave myself time and self-compassion. I embraced many inspiring books and bathed in learning and inspiration, building insights that it is possible to make a shift for the better. I realized it is a conscious choice, and that it is possible to release trauma and hidden blockages, creating access to more powerful internal resources.

My gateway to connection

Coming home I took a Neuro Linguistic Programming (NLP) course for my personal growth and I started meditating regularly. Walks in nature, and especially along the sea, became my best friend during my convalescence. The sound of waves striking against the beach became an immediate healing sound, and the ripples of the water became a strong metaphor to how conscious and constant small changes can give healing and stabilizing effects.

The joy of painting and being creative also opened me up to a world of color and seasonal changes in nature, birds singing, listening to music and reading books, which I had unknowingly shut out. NLP also became my entry point and awakened my curiosity to other areas such as positive psychology and conscious communication. I chose to become a certified NLP Coach, started my own company, and left a well-paid and secure job in the corporate world. This was one of my best decisions ever, after starting meditation, being in nature, and letting my creative side flourish.

Practicing meditation every morning and evening gave me the sacred space I needed to stay connected. Being connected to myself and my loved ones gave me a deeper and broader sense of joy and fulfillment as well as the feeling of being stronger.

The survival strategies I developed in my previous years will still possibly emerge in a new costume, but now I am more prepared. I did as well as I could, as you do and as my parents did. And God bless them for that. by changing my beliefs about myself and opening for a future bigger than my previous one, this helped my children to grow up in a more resource-filled environment than I had.

Now I know the things I value the most are genuine self-expression, courage and freedom, where I am approaching life with excitement, and feeling inspired, alive and energetic. I can see and feel myself. I am not perfect. I do not want to be perfect; I want to be caring, loving and authentic. For me, it's about opening to myself, embracing me and my divine self allowing me to continue giving, but also receiving. I value treating people with care, integrity, respect, and love. My vibe is of an easy-going nature, being intuitive and visionary, while noticing and appreciating beauty and excellence all around me. I am feeling most alive, creative and free when I am bringing my "little spark of madness" with me. Overall, my vibe is working silently and invisibly to nurture and sustain life, being creative and curious.

The basic need of human connection

I am sitting here smiling and reading my own words, knowing that life is amazing. I know, due to my own journey, it is possible to make a shift for the better. As part of my commitment and engagement to serve others, and in addition to my daily work, I have chosen to contribute what I can to help others. Each year I offer free coaching to managers in volunteer organizations, plus I volunteer as a mentor for Global Dignity Day.

Deep and genuine connection with myself and others was seemingly what I was searching for. Human connection is the magic that is born out of souls. A lack of deeper connection to ourselves and others left me feeling empty and out of my core – like being a drift in a sea of strangers.

In my experience nowadays, working with a wide assortment of clients, over the last couple of years, I've had various opportunities to help several people who previously experienced setbacks, exhaustion, and depression. I'm happy to report that most of them have made full recoveries from the burnout they once experienced. These issues vary from the pressure of perfection to managing the stress of thinking you're not good enough, to coping with codependency, a lack of fulfilment, job-related issues like overachieving or burden of service, which I typically see in teachers, nurses, coaches, and therapists – just to mention a few.

Never in history have we had so many devices and ways to help us to connect with other people, oddly enough, we have never felt so disconnected from our souls and tribe like we are now. What's missing is the lack of meaningful connections. Lost connections are the root cause of many of our illnesses and grief. Without meaningful connections we often try to squeeze or silence that bitter pain of disconnection by being over-busy, over-eating and drinking, gambling, drugs, sex, computer games, pornography – in fact anything that adjusts our mood in the short term. We try to cover up our pain with coping strategies, but the pain is still there. The way I adapted to unhappy childhood emotions left them bleeding under the surface of my adult self – unhealed and raw.

Maybe you are feeling a little burned out, or you think there's more to the perpetual feeling of tiredness that you've been experiencing. Well, cheer up! There's hope… I can assure you that the opportunities, fulfilment and joy that await you in the future are far greater than the unpleasant feelings that you may be experiencing right now.

If you felt disconnected from love in your childhood, it becomes much more difficult to trust any loving connections as an adult. The testing out of such potential connections often breaks and destroys them, and it left me alone in that familiar pit of lonely misery.

What would I have done if I had not landed on some final, weird me, whom I embraced with all my heart? It would have been sad to give up the quest. And I invite you to do the same. It is possible to make a change for the better. We are wired to connect.

When we are connected, we feel whole, we heal, we grow, we love.

About the Author

Mona Winbrant is a Life Passion Empowerment Coach, Trainer and Mentor. She is dedicated to increase awareness and wellbeing through her personal and professional self-empowerment programs and considers herself a global citizen. She can see potential, possibilities and pathways to create amazing personal transformations visualizing her client's superpowers. Her specialties are conscious communication, positive psychology and neuroscience.

Mona thinks your darkest and most painful moments in life may hold the key to your life's greatest mission. by exposing your most vulnerable self you will become your own greatest gift. She wants you to see what is possible and that you believe that is possible for you as well.

Her wish for you is to shine bright, be free, and move from surviving to thriving in order to create a life of flow, fulfilment and joy.

Mona would love to hear from you.

Email: mona.winbrant@gmail.com

www.MonaWinbrant.com

Facebook: www.facebook.com/MWinbrant

Instagram: @mona_winbrant

Walk Without Purpose
by Lene Kirk

Nature has always meant a lot to me, and since my childhood it has been a big part of my life. Nature is the most precious thing to me. It gives me peace when I need it, energy when I'm tired, and a feeling of inner power and grounding when I'm extremely busy or need to make important decisions. Nature makes me feel alive and gives me the courage to grow.

I feel like I was born on the water. My parents were sailing a lot when I was a child. My life was by the sea, and in the surrounding coastal nature. I was always outdoors, regardless of the weather. Maybe this is the reason I enjoy the changing seasons and nature's elements so much in my life.

I am highly sensitive, have a strong inner power, and I care a lot about other people. That's the reason why it is so important for me to have inner peace and a lot of energy and calm in my body, which gives me a surplus of energy to go around.

My deepest passion is to help other people, and I share gladly from my inner wisdom because I have many tools and great knowledge. I can help people recover their life energy, especially from periods of stress, where they experience low energy, or after a period where they forgot to take care of themselves. I am working with the whole body, brain and heart.

I am no stranger to stress

My passion for caring for people in need has driven me through a very stressful period of my life. A period where I forgot myself. I forgot my faith, my need for nature, my own health care, my body, brain and heart.

As an affiliate consultant to a company that helps others through stress, I was driven into such violent stress that I forgot my own needs. I pushed myself very hard to help others and I got myself wrong. I criticized myself for being weak when I couldn't help other people through their stress, which I otherwise have such success and experience with.

I spent more and more of my private time working for the company. During that period, I forgot all about being close to nature. There was less and less time for me. My creativity disappeared, as did the other guidelines I had for joy of life and excess energy.

All my effective methods of sustaining energy, and grounding disappeared from my life quietly. My days became more and more absorbed by how I could control my day. It was all about surviving.

My to-do lists got longer and longer, my energy level was minimal, and I spent the evenings and weekends with all the administrative tasks. I worked all the weekends too. My business week went from an agreement of 5 conversations per day to 8 conversations per day and from working 3 days a week to 5 days per week. Plus I was teaching and training in mindfulness and mindset.

My heart and knowledge drove me to give and give and, until suddenly it became confusing and my energy disappeared more and more from day to day. My struggle had truly begun. I felt dizzy, often forgot to breathe, and my body became more and more stiff and tired. From being a nature lover, I preferred to be inside my house. Every time I went outside, I got cold. My legs became heavy and tired. Yet I did not feel I could let go of the work agreement, because people needed my help.

With my experience and knowledge of stress — how could *I* get so stressed?

Guilty

With this sense of guilt on my conscience, my creativity disappeared, thus also the joy and care of myself. Throughout my life I have used my creativity and connection with nature as my guideline to know how I feel. But instead, I was more in my head and not in my body. I couldn't feel my body at all. I was confused in everyday life.

One day it was enough

I had not listened to my body and soul for a long time. It felt like I had lost myself because I could no longer concentrate and simply be present. I felt a need to control everything, meaning I always needed a plan. I made huge demands on myself, even without listening to what was good for me.

I had the feeling that I had to move big mountains daily. It was hard and I was tired in my body and soul. There were many nights without sleep, where I just lay in silence and looked at the ceiling in the bedroom. My head was empty. There were no thoughts, no words or dreams.

I stopped feeling. I felt nothing. My body was like a shell.

I had many excuses to continue that way, but one day I woke up with blurred vision. In the beginning, I thought I had got something in my eye, but it stayed there. My vision was completely blurred and the colors became increasingly gray. Several days passed by before I took it seriously. I had now almost completely lost sight in my right eye. It was so blurred that driving a car would be dangerous.

In addition, my body was even more stiff. In fact, I had pain in my legs every time I moved which meant that I needed to take a break from exercise training as well as yoga. The only thing I felt in my body was pain.

There were no more excuses left

My doctor said I needed peace, but it was difficult. I had to get sick leave from the company. It was a hard decision to make.

It was supposed to be me who helped people who were sick or stressed. I consider myself as a very strong person, therefore it was hard for me to stop and recognize that I needed to take a long break where the only focus would be on me. Only me.

When I finally had surrendered to peace, silence and no chores, I lay in bed for several days and had the feeling of not being able to move. I could only lie still.

My body was tired. My brain and heart did not work. I just lay there for many days with the curtains pulled shut. – I was surrounded by darkness through the whole day. I did not want anything. I did not know what I really wanted.

After many days the sign came in a dream

I remembered my dream in the morning, but I did not write it in my notebook. I knew I dreamed the same dream for many nights and it became increasingly clear.

Then it happened.

A voice said to me: *Lene - You need to step up -* **you must walk.** The voice repeated: *Lene, now you have to walk,* **walk without purpose.** I was confused and did not know where this voice came from. I forgot about the voice again, because I still had a difficult time concentrating.

Before stress, I always listened to my inner voice, but I had overlooked this throughout my stressful period. The voice became more powerful and I knew what to do. No doubt.

Lene, now you need to walk, walk in nature without purpose.

It was my inner voice.

I cried. I cried so much. Now it was possible for me to listen again. I got the feeling of being pulled or lifted out of bed. In a short time, I got more light into my life again. It went fast. The more I listened to my inner voice the faster it went. Step by step I got more and more energy back in my body. My sight was getting clearer and clearer. In the beginning it was very slowly and in flashes. I could see more and more light and more colors.

I started walking

In the beginning, it was short trips but just going out into nature without having any kind of purpose, only being and moving slowly. It gave me peace.

I had forgotten, really forgotten nature, which had always been such a big part of my life. Nature was the place where I picked up my energy, strength and vitality, but also inner silence, strength and grounding.

My hikes became longer and longer, several times a week. I'd rather a short walk on those tired days than nothing. It was as if my legs were leading me and slowly my body was recovering again.

The creativity that has always been my guideline in relation to the life energy, returned slowly into my life again. The more creativity I recognized in my life the more energy I got. The joy appeared in small glimpses, and when I observed the joy it stayed a little longer each time.

Walking without purpose became my rescue from stress. Nature recognized me, and the more I walked the more my body woke up and became present. Nature became my friend again. I was awakened and slowly began to live my life.

I could feel how my senses were awakened more and more each day. When I was in nature I started to smell again. The scent from the forest and the sea is very different. The clear colors of nature were very strong, and I appreciated the color nuances again. The colors gave me energy. When I took my daily walks I noticed the flowers, trees and leaves and felt them with my hands. I picked up stones from the beach and could sit for hours and look out over the water without seeing anything but the feeling that I came home to my truth.

I heard the waves from the sea and the leaves from the trees. And best of all - I could taste again. I could taste the nuances of the food whether it was sweet, sour, salty or spicy. All my senses were activated, and my body became more alive again. However, it took time before I had full confidence in my body, and for a long time, I had exceeded my own limits.

My stress was very physical in my body. There were not so many thoughts but a huge turmoil in my body.

Moving my way

'Walk away from stress' was like a mantra that told me that every step I took, I was releasing a part of my stress. The more steps I walked the less stress I felt. It was the reason why I bought a pedometer, so I could see how much I let go of stress every day. I could feel every day how I was almost pulled outside.

I started my yoga practice again; developing my own silent and relaxed yin practice to work on my body and mind deeply. I started listening to the silence and to the signals I got from my body.I often practiced yoga in my garden, so I automatically felt that nature backed me up. Nature was my support and became my friend again.

My creativity returned

The happy and spontaneous Lene came back in glimpses at first, and then suddenly became a part of me again. Today I see very clearly. And I knew that all kinds of development were happening throughout my entire body before it worked again, because the body remembers everything. Letting go of stress – step by step - helped me to recover.

Today I live in flow with the elements of nature and the seasons. My focus is on the elements in my life and in all my teaching. I especially help women to regain joy of life through training with the body, brain and heart - where nature and the elements help to strengthen the grounding and inner power.

Stress has taught me how important it is to take care of myself and be grateful to have nature as the foundation in my life. I discovered that when I forgot all about the nature and creativity, I lost myself. I have learned how important it is to take a break and be in silence. Every day.

I am even more aware of nature's flow, which helps to create a natural balance in my life. When you follow the flow, you follow the inner and outer development. Everything is energy; - both colors, relationships, objects, nature, and our surroundings, and what we create with our mind, but only when we are present.

The more I am in balance with the seasons and the elements in my life, the stronger I feel. I noticed how important it is for others to live in flow with nature and the elements too. The seasons change and the strength of nature's elements change too, so you feel the difference in your energy levels. by living so much adapted to the season, we naturally get the absolute best tools to get strengthened throughout the year. But it only works when we listen.

I forgot to listen to my body and lost myself and nature's strength. It was there all the time, but I had moved the focus away from myself and to all others.

"Putting the focus from my mind into my body makes a world of difference".

Every single day I am grateful for my contact and connection with nature, and it is an important guide for me.

It gives me strength and life energy. Nature will support you and me in everything.

It sounds easy: "**Walk without purpose**" but it was my challenge and my big adventure to gain renewed zest for life.

I found my way by being with nature, and perhaps it could help you too.

About the Author

Lene Kirk is a passionate Transformational coach, teacher, energy mentor and lightworker from Denmark. She has developed a special kind of yoga called silent yin and silent relaxation for highly sensitive people.

Lene has a private practice offering transforming communications for women and highly sensitive people, yoga and mindfulness training combined with nature, courses, workshops and retreats.

Lene inspires women to rediscover the life energy and joy of life after stress, trauma or other life circumstances. She also provides coaching for sensitive people to train their mindset, habits, and their bodies to feel their inner power and how to connect with nature.

Lene believes you have the possibility for work with your consciousness in a deep way by listening to your heart, mind and body. Lene's passion is to use nature as a strength to live a happy life in every season.

For more information on her programs and services, please connect with Lene.

Online: www.mindmentor.dk

Facebook: www.facebook.com/lene.kirk

Email: hey@mindmentor.dk

Telephone +45 28812700

Tips to Create Positive Connections

During the stressful times of your life, resist the temptation to withdraw into a cave. Instead, give yourself 'permission' or a 'prescription' to connect with positive people at least once per week, if not more. This can act like a lifeline for you when times are tough, and when things are going well, it can be lifeline for your friends.

You don't want to waste time, but staying connected to either discuss your problems or to at least get a break from your own drama can help you. It is incredible how much better we often feel by a change of environment and an opportunity to talk about normal things as well as what is troubling us.

If you don't feel like talking, going for a walk in nature with a friend is a wonderful way to walk off tension and connect without feeling the need to talk about your problems. Being outside will also ground you, shift your stagnant energy, fill your lungs with fresh air and energize you and your friend.

When you can connect with people who are uplifting or supportive of you, you will bounce back faster. Positive people have the ability to make you feel as though a load has been lifted from your shoulders, because they believe anything is possible and they will champion you too.

List at least 3 people you can count on for uplifting conversation and nonjudgmental support.

What is it you love about them?

How do you feel when you spend time with them?

How can you show them how much you appreciate them?

If you are seeking more positive people in your life, the following tips will help you to be the lighthouse that brings positive people towards you:

Keep it real — show up as yourself and don't worry about people who don't like you or 'get you'. Friendships built on authenticity are the most precious gifts we can give each other

Give as much as you get — what can you offer others, how can you brighten their day or make them smile?

Shine a light on them — take time to notice others and really see them. Tell them when they look amazing, or comment on how bright their eyes are.

Be interested, not just interesting — ask people questions about themselves and really listen to what they have to share. People are fascinating when you peek under the surface

Transmit positive vibes — learn to see the lighter side of life and share this liberally with others. There is enough toxicity in the world, so send out positive vibes to offset them

Respect your differences — we all resonate with different things. You can have delightful friendships with people from all walks of life when you celebrate and respect the differences between you.

Smile at strangers — have you noticed how often you receive a smile back when you smile at someone? Smiling at others from a genuine place of connection opens your heart and draws people to you. You can enhance someone else's day with a simple smile.

Resilience Trait #9
Positive Emotion

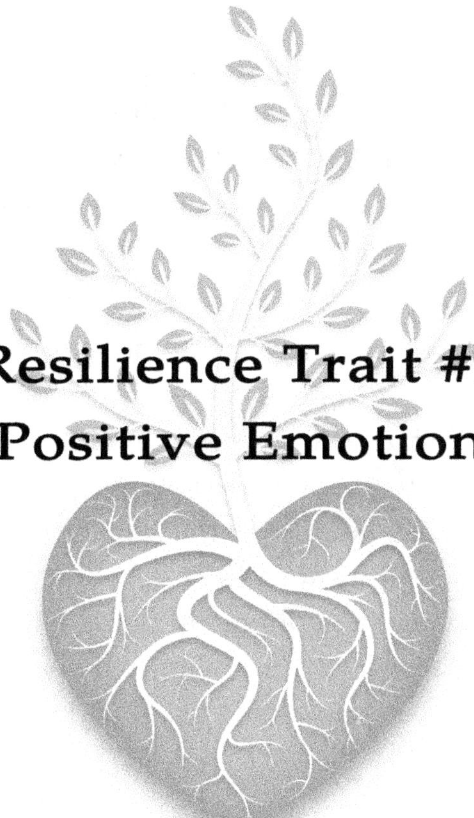

Experiencing joy, gratitude, amusement and awe have been proven to help us build resources to deal with life's many challenges and negative emotional experiences. According to positive psychology researcher Jennifer Stellar, awe-inspiring experiences profoundly impact our physical and mental health.

Experiencing positive emotions opens our hearts, elevates our state, makes us feel inspired and helps us to bounce back from difficult circumstances. Even the simple act of smiling positively impacts our system, because it signals the body to release neurotransmitters such as endorphins, and this elevates our mood.

Positive emotions shift your nervous system from the sympathetic (fight or flight) state, to the parasympathetic (rest and digest) state. When you are relaxed, you slow down, take more in and your peripheral vision expands. Research shows that because of this, positive emotions literally expand your awareness of the wider world. This helps you to be more accepting and more in tune with the needs of other people, which explains why shared joyful experiences transcend boundaries and make us feel deeply connected with each other.

Have you noticed that when you feel joyful, you are better at pivoting and adjusting when life doesn't go as planned? This is because when you feel stressed, you have less tolerance for unexpected changes and reduced capacity for solution-focussed thinking.

The practice of gratitude is scientifically proven to boost positive emotions and help you to process difficult emotions more easily. Gratitude also helps you to sleep better and live longer, as well as boosting your sense of self-worth. Dr. Martin Seligman, the founder of Positive Psychology, studied almost 600 people after they adopted one of five activities designed to boost happiness for a period of one week. He discovered that the most impactful practices were writing down great things that happened that day and expressing gratitude in the form of a gratitude letter.

The most staggering aspect of this study was that when participants who were followed up six months later, they were still much happier than before they started the study, even though they only did one week of daily gratitude practice. This is because starting a gratitude practice sends a message to our brain to start looking for the positive aspects of life, so even when you are in potentially stressful situations, you respond in a more positive way.

If you want to develop your resilience, perhaps by starting a gratitude practice, there are several suggestions in the tips section to help you boost your mood and celebrate life rather than fight with it. If you do start your own regular positive practice, you will also experience the side effects of being more likable, more considerate of others and more appreciative of the relationships in your life.

If this seems like too much of a stretch, picture people in the public eye who have overcome adversity and emerged with a smile on their face. The people you picture will generally be the ones that already inspire you, so ask yourself what it is about them you like, and see how you can embody more of that quality too.

The story shared in this chapter by Sarah K Brandis, provides insight into how escaping the pattern of negative thinking and unconsciously driven 'doing' can lead to positive emotions. This is no trivial pursuit, as Sarah's story shows us. Once we start savoring the good things in life and deliberately generating positive emotions we transform who we are. If you've had a stretch of many years — or decades — of being numb to your feelings, or only having bad feelings, this story will show you a gradual path to more resilience through tuning into positive emotion.

The 'Doing' Trap and Learning to Feel
by Sarah K Brandis

People like to introduce themselves with a title, something that sums up what they do and gives a first impression without too much explanation. Here are a couple I use:

"I'm a marketer."

"I'm an author."

Now there's another one I sometimes use, particularly when asked about my family:

"I'm an elective orphan."

I chose this title for myself because, as us Brits love to say, "It does what it says on the tin."

It explains where my family is – and the honest answer is, "who knows," followed by a shrug and a change of subject. It explains my situation in a heartbeat, without things getting too complicated, and without too much of that social awkwardness.

At the time of writing I have been an elective orphan for 21 years, and to put your mind at rest, I've never doubted my decision once.

My family situation was toxic from a very young age – and for my parents too. I'm sure that their relationship was toxic from long before I joined them. My father was the angry, intimidating type, but often he could get his way just by being in the room – he rarely had to use physical force.

On the other hand, my mother was hands-on violent with me constantly. I always felt that she was afraid of my father, and was kicking downward, venting her frustration at me, the eldest child.

I spent most of my teenage years plotting my escape, then a few months before turning 17 I finally executed my plan and made a break for freedom. It was the bravest, most terrifying and biggest leap ever, and I couldn't have made a better call for myself. The thing about toxic relationships is that when we stay in them, we are the victim forever.

There comes a point where you have to claim your power, focus on what you can control rather than what you can't, and do what's right for you.

The thing about doing what's right for you is that the *'doing'* part can become a negative pattern too. Just like when I was stuck in a victim pattern, controlled by my parents, I later controlled myself with my 'doing' pattern.

Freedom, meet responsibility

I will explain what I mean soon, but let's start where my life truly began. No, not the day I was born, but almost 17 years later, the day that I left the family home for good.

I think for any teenager, suddenly being one hundred percent responsible for yourself would be overwhelming. Personally, I didn't have a clue how to look after myself. I had been so controlled, I didn't even know how to use a can opener as in my mother's house I wasn't supposed to touch things in the kitchen.

The first few years of my new life were purely about learning to survive. I focused on my life just one week at a time; keeping a roof over my head, finding ways to feed myself on my tiny budget from the low-paid jobs I worked, and trying not to be located by my parents.

Although my father had taken my running away as a huge insult and returned the sentiment by declaring me ex-communicated from the family, it was a different story for my mother. She would keep turning up at my accommodation or at my places of work, trying to convince me to come back to her house of horrors.

Just incase you are wondering if putting my story out into the world puts me at any risk of her turning up in my life again, then don't worry, it doesn't. Brandis isn't my family name. I changed my name by deed poll when I was 21. This seemed to solve the problem of her looking me up, and it also meant I got a cool name. I chose Brandis because it means 'fire sword'.

Who wouldn't want to be named after a flaming weapon? I got the documents through the post, and immediately felt like more of a badass.

So it took me a few years to find my feet and even to find a real sense of self. As I had been controlled for so long, it really felt like I was starting from scratch, creating a whole new me.

But once I was ready, the *'doing'* began.

Coming from such a rocky start in life, I was really keen on making something big of my life. I wanted to prove that not could I live without my parents, but also that I could thrive, do better without them – even prove that I WAS better than them. It would be fair to say I had a bit of a chip on my shoulder.

But you know, back then I wasn't very spiritually enlightened. I thought only the end result mattered – not my motivation for why I was pushing for growth and achievement.

My 'doing' list so far…

So do you want to hear what I got up to over the next 15 or so years of my doing campaign? Okay, but just to warn you, it is a bit of a brag list.

In the years since I left home, I have:

- Changed my legal name by deed poll
- Had cosmetic surgery
- Moved across the country many times and briefly worked abroad
- Pole danced at some high-end Gentlemen's clubs
- Managed a central London live music venue and met a lot of famous bands
- Got a tattoo down the entire length of my spine
- Got married, and then swiftly divorced
- Ran the New York Marathon, without coaching or any help
- Ran several more full marathons

- Studied Neuroscience at University of Westminster, while holding down another very cool job and writing my first book for self-publication
- Made the leap to self-employment as a content marketer and writer

I could go on a bit more, but I'm already sounding like a huge bragger. In all honesty I didn't do all this stuff to brag about it to others. I promise I don't stand in my local pub telling everyone I meet that I run marathons or worked with rock stars. I did all these things to try and feel good about myself, to feel like I was somebody worthwhile, and to prove that I could do better without my parents.

Spoiler alert - it never really worked,

After all this stuff on the list, I still didn't feel good. To be honest, I only ever felt negative emotions, such as the feeling I hadn't done the things well enough.

When I crossed the finish line of the New York Marathon, I felt really disappointed in myself. Sure, I had finished the course, but I hadn't done it in the ludicrously naïve time goal I had set myself. So I felt bad for a while, and then I went numb. This felt like unfinished business, and that has a lot to do with why I went on to run more marathons. I just couldn't scratch that itch and do things 'well enough' to feel happy or proud.

I wondered if I ever would get there.

It turned out that yes I would, but not in the way I expected. I would feel happy, satisfied, and proud of myself.

And even better than that, I would stop overachieving to prove something to myself about being better than where I came from. I would start doing things because I felt passion for them.

Hold tight, I'm getting to that part of the story...

What goes up must come down

Of course, like with any good story, I had to hit rock bottom before I could fully learn my lesson and gain the level of understanding I needed to break my old pattern of doing.

It turns out I'm a classic example of somebody who burns out. In my old pattern I had two speeds; stop and go. In a 'stop' period I was depressed. I first experienced this at the age of 22 when burning the midnight oil in a bar job combined with working dayshifts in a fast food restaurant led to me crawling into bed and not coming out for months.

After a few bumbled attempts at recovery and an adverse reaction to Fluoxetine, a particularly tricky antidepressant, I bounced back, determined never to crash like that again.

But it wasn't the things that had caused me to get into bed for months to begin with that I was determined not to repeat – I had pretty much forgotten I'd even worked myself that hard. It was the depression I intended never to repeat.

So knowing that my 'stop' speed took me to the land of nothingness, feeling hopeless and living under a duvet, I focused on my other speed. Go.

Go mode

Going through life in go mode was crazy. It's how I got through that list of achievements above – but it was also what kept me from feeling.

So far in life I had done negative emotions, depression and dark thoughts under the duvet. I had done hopelessness and resentment back at my parent's home. I had done fear when I first stepped out into the world alone and claimed my freedom.

Now I was doing numb.

The amount of work I took on kept me out of the danger zone for depression, but it also kept me from smelling the flowers, feeling the sun on my face, and all of that good stuff.

It was only a few years ago that I crashed and burned my way out of this pattern. I stopped because I had to, but I'm really glad that happened to me.

Of course, there was a big, pivotal moment of awakening. *You didn't think I was going to leave you without one, did you?* Mine came at a work event, which was a little inconvenient. I mean, you don't ever want to cry uncontrollably at a work event, right?

Three years ago, when I had only just started working at Make Your Mark Global with Dr. Andrea, I was attending my first Speak From The Heart workshop as a fairly new part-time team member. Sitting at my desk in the back corner of the room, trying to hide behind my laptop, I couldn't stop the tears running down my face.

I had been listening to one of our speakers, Deri Llewellyn-Davies, talking about his passion for adventuring, among the other aspects of his life, such as business and family. I was really struck by how 'wrong' I suddenly realized I had things. I became aware all at once that I had been numbly ploughing through and pursuing endless work goals for so long that I had forgotten to enjoy anything that I was doing.

I looked at my work schedule, a multi-colored spreadsheet of names and jobs. I had 14 clients on the go, every week on a regular basis. It was no wonder I had stopped feeling, it was the only way to keep going. As I sat there with tears rolling down my face, and really undoing the professional look I had dressed for that day, I started drafting an apology letter to the clients I now knew that I had to let go of.

I was burnt out and miserable — I just hadn't felt it until now.

A whole new world

Now that I can feel joy, and happiness, and all those good things, I am in a much better place mentally. I have to look back and think about what I was meant to learn from this experience. For me, it seems that it all had a lot to do with fear.

When I paused long enough to listen to what the world wanted to teach me – I started to finally understand. All the achievements in the world are nothing if you can't feel them. I needed to learn to feel positive emotions. I had to stop being scared to let them in, in case they made me soft or less ambitious. I had to stop being afraid of resting, standing still and listening. I had to trust that feeling good wouldn't leave me vulnerable to a toxic person like my mother swooping in and stealing my happiness.

As I listened to my thoughts unravel, I realised that I had been so tightly clenched all this time because I was afraid. The 'lesson' or 'truth' I had learned in my house of horrors family home was that joy was there to be stolen, snatched away, and all that I deserved was misery. I had to unlearn this.

Although it's now been 21 years since I physically set foot over my mother's threshold, I had been mentally trapped there for most of my 'free' adult life.

Isn't that funny? How someone can be physically uncaged but mentally still stuck in their prison… But this is what I had to understand before I could change. I had to know that it is safe to feel positive emotions.

Not only is it safe, but it is essential if you want to be a happy, resilient, present person. Please take it from me – nobody can rob you of happiness like you can yourself.

Take a moment to let that sink in.

At the age of 38 I have spent more years out in the world, in charge of myself than those 16 years and 9 months I spent living in a controlling, toxic environment. Yet I've only been truly happy for the last few years or so.

Let that sink in too.

At the end of the day it's not really about how much you do or don't do. Obviously there are extremes to watch out for. Do too much and you will burn out. Don't do anything and the lack of purpose will lead to depression. But within the standard range of 'doing', it's not about what you do, but about what you feel.

I started by finding a coach that I trusted to help me talk my way to understanding what I was beginning to realise about my fear of feeling. From there, it was an exercise is feeling one small thing at a time. I still practice this today – pausing for a moment to feel the small, everyday good things, like my cats greeting me at the door, or the smell of a fresh coffee.

Does what you are doing make you feel good? Does it light you up with passion and feel like you are in flow? Great, that's what you want. That's what writing does for me – and not what my old jobs ever did – not that hanging out with bands wasn't cool, but it didn't make me feel those positive emotions in the same way that writing does. When you start feeling, you will soon know what you are here on planet earth to do.

I know what I'm here to do now, and I know what brings me joy. I absolutely love writing, and I know I'm here to share the lessons from my life through this very medium.

I love running – even more so now that I am able to enjoy my runs without scrutinizing my speed or always making it about a specific goal. It's okay to just run and to enjoy it, and when I am in a timed race, I know that my time doesn't define my worth.

I've also discovered a huge love for cats that I didn't know was in me until recent years. Sure, I've always liked them since I was a child, but I didn't really bond with a cat until I was over my 'doing' phase enough to sit still with a cat and appreciate all the wisdom they have to share with us. Seriously, if you need help slowing down or taking better care of yourself, just go talk to a cat. They know what it's all about.

So that's my story of going from doing to feeling – but it's just the end of a chapter, not the end of my learning and growing. Life isn't something you figure out once and then that's the end. We need to wake up and keep learning everyday. The journey is the destination, and the destination is the journey.

About the Author

Sarah K Brandis is Director of Content at In8Vitality and Make Your Mark Global, and Editor of In8Vitality Magazine. Before finding her feet in the world of marketing, she studied Cognitive Neuroscience at University of Westminster, London, and self-published her first book while navigating a career change from pub manager, to student, then finally content marketer.

Sarah lives in London with her partner and their 3 rescue cats. She loves distance running and dreams of completing all the world marathon majors one day.

Follow Sarah on Instagram:

- For her marketing posts @sarah_k_brandis
- For her running posts @runningwithmymind
- And for In8Vitality @in8vitality

Tips for Beating The Blues by Increasing Positive Emotions

As you have discovered in this chapter, experiencing joy, gratitude, amusement and awe help you to build your resources, so that you can deal with life's challenges and negative emotional experiences.

The following tips are all wonderful methods for accessing more positive emotions and shifting negative ones. It is beneficial to let yourself feel your emotions, good and bad, so that you build your resilience by learning how to process them. Sometimes giving yourself permission to cry makes you feel a lot lighter and less overwhelmed. Remember that emotions are just energy in motion, so let them move through you to increase your emotional capacity to feel positive emotions more often.

Many studies conclude that the daily practice of writing in a journal about 3 things that went right in your day, can help you create more gratitude and happiness. As you reflect on these, take time to really feel the good feelings that arise. This opens your heart and increases your sense of satisfaction and fulfillment.

My family and I enjoy watching inspiring TED talks to remind ourselves that our problems are small and that there are many ways to overcome the blues. Some of the speakers make you feel incredibly lucky and it is humbling to watch them and hear about their work and passions.

Some people enjoy watching videos of baby animals doing funny or heroic things to bring a sense of wonder, delight and awe back to their day. Even watching nature documentaries can be awe-inspiring, as you take in phenomenal scenery and marvel at our incredible planet.

Watching comedy films, listening to funny podcasts, or reading a joke a day makes you smile and helps you forget any worries for a while. This boosts your mood and floods your system with happy hormones like serotonin, dopamine and oxytocin.

Hugging someone for at least 10 seconds can provide a feeling of comfort, safety and connection plus gives you a brain boost of oxytocin to help you stay upbeat. Touch is a powerful way of connecting to other humans and also helps you to get out of your head!

Move your body. Go for a walk or a run, or do some yoga. Put on a mood-boosting playlist and dance like no one is watching. This releases feel-good endorphins into your system, shifting stress, boosting your energy and elevating your sense of 'joie de vivre'.

Celebrate small wins. We overlook so many of the small steps we take, focussing only on the ones we didn't take. Sometimes even getting out of bed is a win. Other days you feel like you can climb a mountain. Celebrate it all and remind yourself how incredible you are to show up daily.

Use your tech to support you. We always have our smart phones these days, so use this to serve you. Set a couple of alarms to go off at intervals during the day and change the text to something positive. Use a phrase such as 'time to smile at yourself' or choose words that resonate, such as 'grateful, present, joyful'.

One of my favorites mood boosters comes from wearing a SMILER — a magical instrument of joy created by a beautiful Icelandic artist and author named Gegga whose story is presented in Chapter 4 . Inspired by a quote by Thich Nhat Hanh she created a little helper that when put into your mouth makes you smile.

"If you smile five times per day for NO REASON, you can change your life in 90 days."

So whatever tool you use, find a reason to smile or experience awe and wonder several times each day.

Resilience Trait #10
Purpose + Meaning in Life

Why do you get up in the morning? What is it that gives your life meaning? Do you feel a sense of purpose in what you are doing?

Having a purpose to live for, or what the Japanese call "Ikigai" has been clinically shown to correlate with less stress-related disease and longer life. In Okinawa in Japan, home to some of the longest-living people in the world, there is no word for retirement. The Okinawans honor their Ikigai daily and it is their reason to get up each morning.

Part of the reason purpose is helpful for our health is that it causes changes in the brain that allow us to adapt to stress. Purpose in life is linked to improved prefrontal brain function and better adaptability to changing situations. Studies show that connecting with a purpose beyond mundane life can help you reduce anxiety and aggression following stressful events.

Cultivating a sense of purpose comes naturally to some people and seems like an indulgence to others, but without it, we tend to wither and lose interest in life as it ceases to have meaning.

Humans are teleological, which means we're naturally wired to move towards targets. It keeps our brains engaged, expands our thinking and gives us a sense of how our daily activities contribute to the bigger picture. Without purpose it can be hard to fight the urge to stay in bed every morning. What gets us up is the inner knowing we have to contribute in some way.

Our teleological drive also points to our capacity to find more fulfillment when we focus on contributing to something far bigger than ourselves. This capacity is a key factor to developing resilience, as when we are dedicated to service rather than satisfaction, we are strongly incentivized to keep going, even when we want to give up.

Your sense of meaning may come from a tangible, measurable activity or aim, or it may arise from a deeper sense of connection to your more esoteric spiritual side. Studies have shown that those who are more spiritual tend to be more resilient as well. This may be because people with a strong sense of spirituality feel supported by an energy bigger than themselves, or it could be due to the connections this fosters in their lives.

Spiritual meaning does not have to be esoteric. It can also come from regular excursions in nature, a dedicated yoga practice, love of surfing, women's circles or other meaningful pursuits. The whole point of finding meaning and purpose is to find something that fills you up, because when you have inner fulfillment and intrinsic happiness, you no longer rely on external circumstance to dictate your state.

Think about what brings you the biggest sense of fulfillment in your life. What brings a smile to your face when you remember it? Is there an activity you do regularly that you would happily do for the rest of your life? What or who lights you up and can you identify the reason why?

Our final story in this book is a truly epic and incredible story about how being connected to a deep sense of purpose helped the author dig deep and find the resilience he needed, when all the odds were stacked against him on

Mount Everest. Prior to developing his sense of adventure and purpose, Deri Llewellyn-Davies was working hard in a job he liked, but he felt trapped on the hamster wheel of life. Following two huge life blows, he shares how he started extricating himself from this life and embarking on a more meaningful path. This powerful story consolidates each chapter in this book in a relatable way, giving you the context for how each one interweaves with the others to make you hugely resilient.

Purpose-led Resilience
by Deri Llewellyn-Davies

Resilience, I believe is built, crafted, and shaped moment by moment, over many years. And it's powered by purpose.

I also believe that "life is a great adventure". Adventure itself just so happens to be one of the core elements of my life, and is the title of my first book. However when I talk about adventure from here on in please substitute YOUR greatest calling whether that is art, yoga, sports or gardening (I like that one, too).

I think deep down a lot of us desire to live a great life. We have a desire to do more, to have more, to be more, and to truly find our purpose. But life isn't filled with magic fairy dust. There is a common delusion many buy into that says when everything is in place, one day, all will be rosy. People think they can seek "happiness" or "joy" or "fulfillment" and upon finding it, somehow it will be the permanent emotion from that point on.

I don't buy that. I once did. But I don't now.

Don't get me wrong, by building that kind of life you should experience way more positive feelings than negative, however what most people aren't preparing you for is what happens when adversity strikes, when those bad moments come. It's how you deal with the crappy times that will define the good times. That's resilience and it needs to be built.

A great life needs to be architected. A full, rich and complex life does anyway. If you seek a simple life I honor you. I sometimes think of what a beautiful existence it would be as a monk, tribesman, or nomad. However, I have chosen a different life, I seek depth in my life, I seek travel, I seek adventures, deep relationships with those closest to me. I love properties and architecture and my homes and gardens, I love nature and I love business. I don't want to give it up and be a monk, yet. I seek it all, all life's great experiences, all life's rich tapestry. And if I want it all I have found I need to architect it.

I cover this concept of architecture within a body of my work called Diamond Life Design, so I won't go deeper here on it. Visit www.DiamondLifeDesign.com for more.

I can say categorically I haven't met anyone who appears to have it all that hasn't consciously designed it, though appearances can be deceiving. I also haven't met anyone who found it all rainbows and fairy dust on that journey. No one finds only experiences of beautiful emotions, feelings of love, joy and happiness.

Now don't misunderstand me here, there have been tonnes of amazing emotions, and feelings along the way, and we can absolutely architect many many more, and we can get massively high percentage of ours lives in the amazing zones of high energy, high feeling. However if we don't learn to manage ourselves when the shit storms come, when the destructive feelings kick in, when you're on your knees, that's when we will quit. That's when we settle. That's when we don't drive forward to the dream, but rather when we retreat to safety and mediocrity. And to get through the storms of life, you need courage, you need to master your emotions, master your mind, and develop resilience.

I always like to get to the basics and to the essence of things quickly, so what is resilience? According to the dictionary it is "the capacity to recover quickly from difficulties; toughness."

So is it a trait we are born with? Or do we learn this? Well by definition if we never put ourselves in tough situations, if we never stretch or don't face difficulties then, no, we won't develop resilience. Now life has a funny way of throwing some stuff at you that you didn't ask for, but if it's only once in a while you are more likely to break than develop resilience.

So resilience is like a muscle built over time by consistent use. The more I push, the more I strive, the more failure I face, and the more tough times I ride through the more resilient I become. Becoming resilient in one area of life can bleed into all areas of life, but again this is best done consciously and architected.

I was on stage in Stockholm, Sweden, and during the Q&A portion at the end of my presentation a lady asked, "what do you define as mastery?" It was one of those "success" audiences who are usually hyped by positive thinking and not mentioning any dark side. And I responded quite flippantly and unprepared;

"It's being in the middle of a shit storm in life, having no idea what to do, having no way out, and not able to see how this can possibly benefit you, and being able to remain centered and calm, with strong inner hope and faith, that all will be ok."

But what trait drives someone to have that kind of mastery, that kind of resilience? I propose that it's living from a strong sense of purpose.

Let's be honest, living life fully in all areas is not an easy thing to do. So many people say to me, "Yes, but I don't have discipline, or money or time" or some other excuse. And I always respond the same way, the only thing you're lacking is a burning desire and a massive purpose. When you have those, nothing can stop you!

I really do get that we are all under pressure from different commitments whether they may be from work, family, financial constraints or the many stressors of life. As such, the things we would REALLY love to do with our lives go to the bottom of the list, and remain a fantasy. For you to step up and prioritise, your WHY needs to be massive. With out that, it will be a fad and it won't last. Like the way diets and the use of gym memberships don't stick.

Nearly 15 years ago, when I began this great adventure that I am now playing full out, I was on the hamster wheel, the rat race, the corporate ladder. I was working hard in a career and whilst it wasn't a big bad career and I wasn't miserable in my job, I had become trapped. I kind of liked what I did; there was no disillusion with what I was doing, I was good at business and was going up the ranks quite rapidly. But that is how things can become a one-track journey.

I was working ridiculous hours, commuting a long distance, working in the city and living to social excess. I had always played rugby but had suffered an injury and had lost a lot of my fitness. I was overweight, my health had gone, my relationship was volatile and my soul was on burnout – there was something massively missing, there was something I was yearning for, something deep.

To find purpose you have to start by going deep and looking inside to find out what the piece is that is missing for you. I think most of us are yearning for something, searching and pondering the inevitable questions such as, "what are we here for?" and "what is it all about?" Ultimately we want to know, "what is our purpose in life?" I believe it's not just one thing, our life purpose shows up in multiple dimensions. And it begins inside, not outside.

I had come to the point where I didn't recognise myself and didn't know who I was. Shortly after I was hit by two intense blows, the end of my rugby career and the death of my father. I think a lot of us don't make tough life decisions when we could or should; it takes something catastrophic in our lives to nudge us in the right direction. For me that was certainly the case, and the death of my father was ultimately what made me think and led me to live purposefully.

My father was a great man and a great influence in my life. Like many of us that have lost someone to cancer, it happened really fast. In the weeks that followed his death, what struck me the hardest was that my father had died without fulfilling his dreams.

This sticks with me, and I think it will continue to stick with me until the day I die.

My father confided in me during the last days of his life that he had been a fool and that he regretted not going out there and doing what he wanted in life. He always said he was going to do this, he was going to that, he was going to travel, he was going to do this with my mum – and he never did, it was always tomorrow, someday or whenever. And Someday isn't in the calendar.

When your father admits he thinks that he has been a fool, had massive regrets and that he was dying with his dream intact, it makes you sit up, shut up and get shit done. That was the point where I decided 'I'm going to live a life of great adventure, with no regrets'. But this meant that I had to be prepared to make tough decisions along the way because living a life with no regrets is not the easy path. I was resilient in business, no doubt, as I had pushed and risked there, but I hadn't translated that muscle into other areas of my life.

I started by exploring myself. "Know thyself," was good enough for the Oracle of Delphi so I figured it was a good place to start. After much personal exploration and evolution with great teachers such as Tony Robbins, John De Martini and Brendon Burchard, I realized something was missing. It was a visualisation of a future me, an older me, with my grandchildren sitting on my knee (at this point I didn't even have kids) and I realised I had nothing to say. I imagined saying how Granddad did these big business deals but talking them through business acquisitions didn't really fit. That's when I saw part of my bigger purpose, my BIG WHY, Adventure...

I always wanted to be an adventurer, but figured that was for some other super breed of a person, not an average guy like me. What BS and what crappy excuses!? Then suddenly I saw life for what it was, a great adventure, nothing less.

When I say adventure, at that point in my life I had decided to say 'screw it', if I'm going to go for adventure I was going to go big. I wanted to experience the best the world has to offer and really explore this wonderful world we live in.

This lead to my Bucket List which I have dubbed "The Global Adventurer's Grand Slam" which included the 7 Summits (The Highest mountain on each of the 7 continents), the 2 poles, the Marathon Des Sables (6 marathons back to back across the Sahara carrying everything you need to survive on your back), the jungle Marathon (6 Marathons across the Amazon jungle) and an IronMan thrown in to the mix! No one had done it before in that context, so I was going for a bit of a world first and that's where the journey began. It started with just a mere dream, as all things do, and then I went to work.

The thing your have to be prepared for when you step into your purpose is that not everyone will feel like you do about what you want to do and you might not get the support you imagined getting. Not everyone dear to me supported me, my mother, God bless her, who supported and was an inspiration to me throughout my childhood was positively anti everything I did (and still is), because they're such dangerous feats. You will need resilience here.

Also before you think I am some super human, then nope, I played rugby in the forwards, was 17 stone and could run well over 20 yards, usually into someone. I am asthmatic, and flat footed. So I needed a lot of resilience mentally to step forward from this decision.

As I write this I am very proud to say I have now completed the Marathon Des Sables, The IronMan and 6 of the world's highest mountains, cumulating in an epic attempt on Everest.

But along this journey things will hit you, things wont go your way, you will face your fears, and this is when you need resilience the most. But purpose is what holds you steady. I think my epic on Everest probably is the greatest metaphor for this.

So imaging you're on Everest, you are fully prepared. Over 10,000 hours of work has gone into that mountain, you have scaled 5 of the 7 summits already, you are ready, you are prepared, you are fit. Everything in your control. That's where I was in 2015.

I was on the final route to advanced base camp (ABC) on the north side of the mountain. It was the Biggest day so far, this was THE PUSH. We were starting the day at 5900m, already at the dizzying heights of Kilimanjaro, where people end their journey, and pushing to 6500m and advance base camp. Each step now was a labour, and we were all sucking in the oxygen hard up there.

We soon got onto a main Rongbuk glacier, and the slog began proper.

We were all just getting on with our own mental activity. As soon as we got on the glacier, we split a little. The front party went ahead, composing of former British Special Air Service and the elite parachute regiment. The back party lingered a bit, with the videographer taking advantage of the beauty and the amazing day and I kinda pitched in the middle on my own. I needed thinking time alone.

The valley was immense, awe inspiring… and was framed each side by magnificent penitentes, the massive 100-200 foot high ice pinnacles. Such awe, such wonder.

The Rongbuk glacier is like the biggest ice sculpture in the world. Designed and built by mother nature; the views of the glacier and the Himalayan peaks are some of the most dramatic in Tibet. And right along the middle moraine of the glacier is a rough trail that weaves across the back of the beautiful beast.

It was a beautiful day and the skies were blue... Then the world moved.

I was on my own, immersed in my own thoughts and my own mental battle. I stopped for a drink and some food. I swung my pack off my back and as I was about to place it on the ground the ground moved from under me so violently it knocked me from my feet.

Suddenly I was riding a bucking bronco and to lose would mean I would be thrown from the face of the earth. I laid down spread eagle on the ground. And grabbed the rocks to hold on. I gripped and held on for dear life.

My mind was racing now, what was going on? Am I having a dizzy fit, has my mind succumbed to altitude and is this HAPE? (High Altitude Pulmonary Edema plus swelling of the brain)?

No. It felt too extreme, too real. Perhaps the whole glacier is moving. Shit, the glacier is on the move! No, this is too violent.

Just hold on Deri – hold on.

Then after about a minute the movement eased and then stopped.

I still hung onto the ground for dear life, drawing blood.

And then there was nothing but total silence. A void in the very fabric of the atmosphere.

Then it began.

For any mountaineer the biggest fear above any is an avalanche. And now just seconds after the greatest mountain on earth had been shaken like a rag doll, the avalanches began. It began like a thunder, a deep rumble like the very bowels of the earth is moving. But in this case there wasn't just one, there were avalanches happening all around.

The entire Rongbuk valley avalanched.

Then the cracking and splintering sounds as the ice penitentes started to crack and smash, 200 ft high. Each side of the glacier. Armageddon was happening all around. And yet there I was, sat upon the glacier, raised above it all, on the only safe part of the mountain, witness to it all. In the palm of God. Witnessing the raw power of mother earth.

I stayed where I was, witness to the continuing rumblings, thunder all around and cracking. Until many minutes later the sounds subsided and there was an eerie silence again. There I sat, stunned, confused and shockingly present.

I felt dizzy, slightly sea sick after riding the wave, slightly unsteady on my feet. So I sat, I drank and I ate, and I waited.

I was waiting for my colleagues to catch up to see if they had any more insight than me. And to reaffirm that what just happened wasn't in my mind, I was still questioning if high altitude had taken its toll and I had gone mental. 15 minutes must have passed until they came over the ridge in front. And they were soon approaching, saying "s***! What was that??!! That was mental…." And yet still not of us had registered what indeed it was.

So after some chat and swapping of war stories on how wild the ride was we needed to crack on, we still had a long way to go. We couldn't sit there and cry and mope; we had to carry on. We were there for a purpose. We had to move and we did.

Resilience

The next part of the day was brutal, and over 4 hours later we finally got to ABC.

I have never been so happy to get to camp. We had done it and there right in front of us was the mother goddess herself, Everest, and the north col. A place of legend and of my dreams for years. A euphoric moment as I breathed in the crisp cold air of the col.

Then the euphoria was to be shattered.

We had no idea quite what we were in. But after a satellite phone call back to the real world, it became apparent that we were in the epicenter of what was turning out to be one of the biggest earthquakes to hit the Himalaya for over 100 years. Already many had died in Nepal, and some of our comrades had died on the south side of the mountain. We would subsequently find out that over 9000 people died that day, and 19 climbers making it the worst death toll on Everest ever and one of the worst and most devastating natural disasters in human history. And we were in the epicentre of the earthquake, no wonder it was so brutal.

So what do we do?

We were now 6500m up on the north face of Everest. Putting that in context helicopters can't fly that high so there is no rescue. This is where two decades of resilience kicks in.

So now all the points of resilience come into play. Everything you have learnt in this book.

1. Time to take a breath, realize who I am, what I stand for and why I'm here. Work I had done for years in meditation.

2. Time for flexibility, all plans as we knew them meticulously worked out are now out of the window. Rigidity won't help us now. Time for plan B.
3. Time to be adaptable, really adaptable. As there was no precedent, no one in history had faced this before.
4. Compassion is now critical for all those dead, for our Sherpas and their families for ourselves, time to dig in deep, really deep.
5. Yet still hold the faith, there is hope, optimism in the face of darkest moment. Now is where positivity is key.
6. Confidence built over 10,000 hours of prep and facing so many adversities on previous mountains.
7. I can do this, this is my time, positive self-talk, built over a decade so the voice is clear and my friend.
8. Team, I have the best in world hand selected.
9. Remember the wonder and the awe at the rawness of Everest. And the blessings of being witness to something so magnificent.
10. Finally purpose.

So I spent 3 days and 3 nights on the north face, a number of my comrades retreated, that left 4 of us. We were in, we were ready, despite a massive set back, this can still be done. Despite the odds, despite the circumstance, fueled by purpose, with a fabric of resilience.

We were eventually forced to retreat by the Chinese authorities, and had to self rescue to get ourselves back to base camp, but that's a longer story. What's important here, is that in that darkest moment, I saw light. I was able to bounce back, was able to clearly make a call to still be fully in, to regroup and confidently and purposefully push on. That mountain was so engrained in my deepest purpose.

That ability was crafted over a decade and continues to build everyday. Resilience is built in the small moments, in every set back we face, how we face every little thing is how we face everything. So face each set back, each fall, each knock, using all the tools in this book. Build day by day moment by moment and when the big tests come you'll be ready. Resilience is your birthright, but like any skill you need to develop it and you can only do so by pushing the boundaries of life, or in my words by living life as a great adventure and being true to your purpose.

About the Author

Deri Llewellyn-Davies is an internationally acclaimed speaker, author, adventurer and entrepreneur who is transforming lives around the world with his core focus on Business, Life Architecture and High performance. Deri shares his love of adventure in his first book, *Life's Great Adventure*, which includes the hidden emotions he experienced as he climbed six of the highest mountains in the world, run the Marathon des Sables, and completed an IronMan. Deri also lived to tell his tale of "No Regrets" after surviving the devastating earthquake while climbing Everest in the spring of 2015 as shared in his hugely popular TEDx presentation.

In a career spanning two decades, Deri's business expertise has included roles on elite corporate boards through four billion dollar companies up to European executive board level. Having run several of his own businesses, advising over 300 boards and speaking to thousands of business owners he brings his audiences deep insights with both a global and local perspective on business and life.

Deri's signature methodologies, outlined in his business book, *Strategy on a Page* and his life architecture model Diamond Life Design, demystify strategic and complex concepts and enable people to gain valuable, practical and actionable principles they can apply immediately.

Visit Deri online at www.Deri.live and check out
Diamond Life Design at www.DiamondLifeDesign.com

Tips to Banish Aimlessness and Find Meaning In Life

It is entirely possible for us all to find a sense of meaning and purpose in life. Purpose and meaning can come from the smallest of things — indulging our hobbies, taking pleasure in walking, enjoying conversations and looking after others.

You can bring a sense of purpose to your existing daily activities just by showing up more authentically and being fully present. Sometimes the meaning we seek is right there under our nose — like learning optimism, it is all about reframing your idea about what meaning has to look like.

A wonderful proactive way to create more meaning and fulfillment in your life is by dedicating some time to a pursuit that gets you out meeting new people and serving a bigger cause.

This opens your heart and makes you feel better about yourself. There is something incredibly powerful about contributing to something far bigger than ourselves and we underestimate how this can improve not only the lives of those we are serving, but also our own.

Explore this by connecting with likeminded people or volunteer for a cause in line with your values. If you can contribute in a way that enables you to fully express yourself, or uses your strengths and talents in service to others, you will increase your sense of meaning and feel a sense of freedom.

The Random Acts of Kindness practice from positive psychology includes doing something nice for someone - ideally a complete stranger - without seeking any recognition or reward. For example, you can put coins into the parking meter of a car you notice has an expired meter, or you can 'pay it forward' to the next customer when you next treat yourself to a coffee.

As an extension of this idea, find a way that you can boost someone else's day by offering them a helping hand, supporting them in some way or maybe sending them a card with a positive message. There are wonderful examples on social media of people leaving random love notes in public places for people to find and even though they will never know who finds them, it is easy to imagine the delight they must feel from doing this each day!

If you feel as though you need more time to be still, so that you can connect with your sense of purpose more often, find a way that you can commit to this by taking one small step. Perhaps you could start a 3 minute meditation practice, or give yourself permission to go for a ten minute walk each day, during which you don't look at your phone and you notice your surroundings. by taking time to yourself on a regular basis, you will nourish yourself and boost your sense of fulfillment.

Having read through these ideas, notice which ones make you feel a sense of hope and possibility. List **one** thing you could do **today** inspired by something you have read, that would make this day worth living.

Conclusion

The stories in this book have probably opened your eyes to new possibilities. They certainly have done that for me. I hope that expanding your mind and exploring new ways to enhance your resilience will become a way of life for you now.

I sincerely wish you an inspired journey in building resilience. If our paths should cross, I hope you will open up and share stories about your own experiences of resilience. Or perhaps you'll do so in one of my upcoming books or a live event?

Feel free to contact the brilliant, brave authors in this book. They are so heart-centered and precious, I know they will inspire you as they have me. Besides, being in the company of amazing people allows their special sauce to rub off on us, and if we let it, their magical qualities can also linger.

Please watch the #AskTheAuthor interview series by visiting and sign up to receive special gifts from the authors.

Many blessings to you,

Andrea and all of the authors of The Top 10 Traits of Highly Resilient People

About the Book's Creator

Dr. Andrea Pennington is an integrative physician, acupuncturist, meditation teacher, and international speaker who is on a mission to raise the level of consciousness and love on our planet. As a personal brand architect, media producer, and communications specialist, she leverages her 20+ years of experience in broadcast and digital media to proudly help healers, Light workers and coaches to bring their brilliance to the world through publishing and media production with Make Your Mark Global Media.

Dr. Andrea is also a bestselling author, international TEDx speaker and documentary filmmaker. For nearly two decades, she has shared her empowering insights on vitality and resilience on the *Oprah Winfrey Show,* the *Dr. Oz Show*, iTV *This Morning,* CNN, the *Today Show*, LUXE-TV, Thrive Global and HuffingtonPost and as a news anchor for Discovery Health Channel. She also produced a four-part documentary series and DVD entitled *Simple Steps to a Balanced Natural Pregnancy.*

Dr. Andrea has appeared in many print publications including *Essence, Ebony, Newsweek, The Sun, Red, Top Santé* and *Stylist.* She has also written or contributed to 12 books. As host of the talk show, *Liberate Your Authentic Self* and as founder of In8Vitality she blends her 'nerdy' mix of medical science, positive psychology, and mindfulness meditation to empower us all to show up authentically, love passionately, and live with vitality.

Visit Dr. Andrea online at:

AndreaPennington.comRealSelf.Love

MakeYourMarkGlobal.comIn8Vitality.com

Get Social!

facebook.com/DrAndreaPennington

twitter.com/drandrea

linkedin.com/in/andreapennington

instagram.com/drandreapennington

Other Books Published by Make Your Mark Global

The Real Self Love Handbook: A Proven 5-step Process to Liberate Your Authentic Self, Build Resilience and Live an Epic Life
by Andrea Pennington

The Ultimate Self-help Book: How to Be Happy Confident & Stress Free, Change Your Life with Law Of Attraction & Energy Healing
by Yvette Taylor

Magic and Miracles
Created and Compiled by Andrea Pennington

Life After Trauma
Created and Compiled by Andrea Pennington

The Magical Unfolding by Helen Rebello

The Orgasm Prescription for Women
by Andrea Pennington

Time to Rise
Created and Compiled by Andrea Pennington

The Book on Quantum Leaps for Leaders: The Practical Guide to Becoming a More Efficient and Effective Leader from the Inside Out by Bitta. R. Wiese

Turning Points
Compiled and Edited by Andrea Pennington

How to Liberate and Love Your Authentic Self
by Andrea Pennington

The Top 10 Traits of Highly Resilient People
by Andrea Pennington

Daily Compassion Meditation: 21 Guided Meditations, Quotes and Images to Inspire Love, Joy and Peace
by Andrea Pennington

Eat to Live: Protect Your Body + Brain + Beauty with Food
by Andrea Pennington

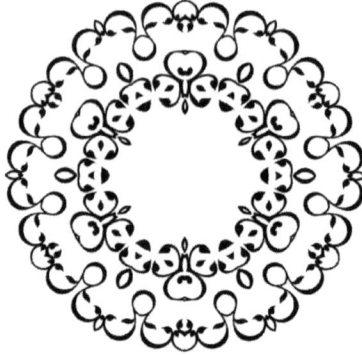

MAKE YOUR MARK GLOBAL

Get Published Share Your Message with the World

Make Your Mark Global is a branding, marketing and media agency based in the USA and French Riviera. We offer publishing, content development, and promotional services to heart-based, conscious authors who wish to have a lasting impact through the sharing and distribution of their transformative message. We also help authors build a strong online media presence and platform for greater visibility and provide speaker training.

If you'd like help writing, publishing, or promoting your book, or if you'd like to co-author a collaborative book, visit us online or call for a free consultation.

Visit www.MakeYourMarkGlobal.com or

Call +1 (707) 776-6310 or

Send an email to Andrea@MakeYourMarkGlobal.com